Hippie at Heart Self-Help Series

THE RETIREMENT
Rebel

How to get your life to work,
when you don't have to

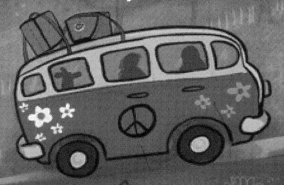

MARGARET NASH

Contents

Introduction

"Many Americans simply don't have a great life in retirement. This chapter of life could be the best and most meaningful, yet far too many experience isolation and a lack of purpose. One symptom of this is that the typical retiree aged 65 to 74 spends four hours per day watching television, according to U.S. News & World Report." –
www.kiplinger.com

Shaquille O'Neal, the retired National Basketball Association champ and one of the most flamboyant personalities in sports history, was recently on the Ellen Show. A giant, clocking in at over 7 feet tall and 300 pounds plus, Shaq is a friendly beast. Ellen asked him if he had any advice for the soon to be retired NBA superstar Kobe Bryant.

"Well," said Shaq, "He's gonna be bored."

"Wait!" cried Ellen. "Are you bored? Don't you have any hobbies? What do you do all day?"

"No, no hobbies. I sit at home, hang out, and watch Ellen."

Now Shaq is obviously exaggerating a bit. He is a popular sports commentator on television and has other activities to keep him occupied. But still, he's making a point.

He's 44 years old, rich and famous, and he's describing the retirement blues.

The Retirement Blues

Retirement! The word conjures up all sorts of images—golf, knitting, bingo, walkers, retirement homes. Not an exciting word no matter how you spin it.

Retirement is when we stop working for a living. For whatever reason—age, income, health reasons, or marrying someone rich—we quit our full time job to do something else Many dread it; others cannot wait. It's scary for some because it involves stepping into the unknown—a brave new world without work to define and structure life.

Retirement can be a huge challenge for many people in a number of ways. Many retirees report that they feel terrific at first, excited and full of plans… and then the blues set in.

The retirement blues spring from the conundrum that when we finally get all the time in the world to do what we want, we don't know what to do with that time.

Isn't it quite shocking how quickly our enthusiasms and passions disappear as soon as we get what we want? How many of us, on that resort holiday, fall madly in love with the quaint little beach town and all those fun shops, local characters, and charming sidewalk cafes? We long to spend the rest of our lives there.

We know with absolute certainty that we would never get tired of lying on the beach, swimming in that crystal clear water, or sipping Margaritas while watching the sunset. But just go ahead and sell your home, up stakes and move there. Put bets on how long it takes before you are tearing your hair out in boredom.

Our dream of retirement can turn out to be one big damp squib.

This damp squib is not the same as depression, more an underlying feeling of unease, restlessness, and disappointment. This is sometimes described as being *in the doldrums*—a state of inactivity, listlessness, stagnation, or low spirits.

A fair description for how we feel when in a transition stage of life, such as retirement, and life is not going as planned. There is no wind in our sails and we feel as if we are drifting on a sea of gloom without an oar.

My journey from England to Houston...and then on to Mexico!

A little bit of background: a decade ago I made the huge decision to move from England, where I had lived for thirty years, to Houston, Texas. If you've been to Houston you will know what I suffered. If you are from there, my sincere apologies. And commiserations.

I should have known better. I come from Alabama, so it's not like it was a foreign country. It was just over the way, past Louisiana, but I had never been there before.

I arrived in Houston, lived in a brain fog for three years, then moved on to Mexico, got remarried, and am living to tell the tale. I have two dogs and a cat. I lost 25 pounds. I'm a couch potato but it's a very nice couch on a veranda draped in bougainvillea and other flowers whose names I don't know. My garden is a wildlife refuge for possum, herons, passing cats, and hummingbirds.

I work as a semi-retired life-coach, writer, and seminar leader. Semi-retired in my case means I dictate when and how often I do anything. It's a nice way to work.

Retirement Blues doesn't even begin to describe what I went through to get here.

So hang in there with me. I may not have all the answers but I have managed to get some things right and I'm willing to share what I have found to work. I may be just a couple of steps ahead of you if you're feeling the blues coming on.

I have strategies. Carefully worked out strategies that saved my life, figuratively speaking. I got my life to work when I didn't have to. Want to know what they are? Read on.

Why this book?

I live in the retirement mecca of San Miguel de Allende in the central highlands of Mexico. Life is slow, relaxed, laid back. People retire here to chill out and enjoy the sociable, easygoing atmosphere, and mild climate. When you arrive you come unglued automatically.

People here look forward to making new friends, having interesting activities, enjoying a new culture, and doing something useful. Charity work? Learning Spanish?

Sounds simple and clear, but many end up watching too much TV or being on the internet more than they care to admit... and the days drift by with nothing much satisfying going on.

And the overwhelmingly persistent chorus from my life-coaching clients is, *I want to find a purpose* and, *I just don't know what to do with myself.*

I translate this: I don't feel ready to be put on the shelf! There's still life in me and I want to express it in meaningful and exciting ways! Help! There's still a kick in my heels and I want to have fun, but also be creative and most of all, relevant. How? *How do I get my life to work when I don't have to?*

This book addresses what Shaq had the nerve to admit – that even when you have everything material in life but lack something compelling to do, then guess what folks? It's afternoon television for you.

Here is a list of common complaints from my retired clients:

- Too many life shaking transitions going on all at once—divorce, empty nest, relocation, at the same time as retiring—and feeling overwhelmed

- Boredom, despite having the time and money to be able to do whatever they want

- Lack of motivation, a feeling of having lost their mojo, no more ambition

- Too much time spent on television and the internet (those who take your computer to bed with you, 'fess up now)

- Missing aspects of their old life, a restless longing for something more.

Does this describe you? It certainly does me. Or did, I should say. I found retirement to be the most challenging time of my life, and I've had a fairly high-octane life. It's been really hard for me to learn how to get motivated and achieve anything meaningful when I don't *have* to.

Retirement in the New Age

"Most people don't want to sit back and slowly decline once they quit working. Many Americans today want to continue to learn and to grow and to share meaningful experiences and interactions with others. They've watched the generation of their parents live out their retirement, and they want something else – something richer and more complex." – www.kiplinger.com

As mentioned earlier, back in the good old days retirement conjured up certain images: the ripe old age of 65, sports and fishing for the men, charity work for the ladies, the game of Bridge as a couple's activity, gentle hobbies, and moving to a sunnier clime such as Florida or Spain. The term was usually associated with men.

Also: old, on the way out, coasting into the sunset, insurance policies, pension plans, savings, health schemes. Nursing homes. Irrelevance.

There was a very clear model to follow. People knew their roles and played their parts and lived out their days in peaceful boredom.

Shoot me now.

Meet the Retirement Rebel

Oh boy, our generation is so different! We are the generation of Retirement Rebels!

Nowadays, for our tribe – new-age-rebel-old-hippie-baby-boomers – instead of Florida and golf, it's Mexico, Bali, or Costa Rica, with art classes, Spanish lessons, yoga and Pilates, and a lot of organic gardening.

We are intrigued by sustainable living, blended communities, communes, retirement villages of all stripe, strange restrictive diets, moving to any foreign country where life is simpler, cheaper, and has more 'culture'. You name it – we're trying it out. We're adventurous if nothing else.

We no longer follow traditional retirement models. We have rebelled against them. Many of us were self employed and had our own businesses. We retire when we please, or when we can afford it. Retirement has now become unconventional; we retire at different ages, with 65 no longer the defined entry point into elderly status. Whew for that!

We like the idea of semi-retirement.

We, the Retirement Rebels, do things our way. We are adaptable, not afraid of change, and not afraid to pioneer. We want to retire and age on our terms and we fiercely resist being told what to do.

Many of us are old hippies at heart and maintain that paradigm busting energy.

We have a plethora of opportunities and loads of resources at our disposal.

Oh, the choice!

But we still get the Retirement Blues! Hmmm...

Picture it. You don't have to work anymore. Wonderful. But even with lots of planning, thinking, dreaming, ticket buying, research, realtors, you simply have no idea what it's going to be like when the time comes and you quit whatever you've been doing to earn a living.

Many report feeling their time on this planet is limited and are in a hurry to get their new lives going: the clock is running out and mortality looms.

Many start to fear death or the loss of loved ones.

But it's not only when friends or family members die that we are affected. When musician Glenn Frey passed away recently I became obsessed with the *Eagles* and couldn't stop playing their music and watching their old videos on YouTube. It's like I wanted to recapture something I had lost in the hazy past of the 70s.

Rock star David Bowie's death caused a frenzy of nostalgia. I was devastated when George Harrison passed on. We get upset when our icons of youth get old and die. They're not supposed to do that. It's uncomfortable to say the least.

The most common fears on retiring are being alone, broke, in ill health, and losing one's looks. The result of these fears can be disturbing. Boomers spend unprecedented sums of money on plastic surgery, which sometimes kills or produces alien look-alikes; they get obsessed about pensions, insurance, savings, Medicare.

There never seems to be enough of anything. They buy burial plots, and join 24-hour societies. Some sink all their money into ill-advised investments, others into retirement villages before being sure it's what they want.

It's always a good idea to be prudent and make sure you can take care of yourself. But obsessive planning won't stave off the retirement blues. It won't keep you from getting bored or feeling out of sorts. It won't give you a sense of purpose.

First world problem?

Let's get this out of the way before we go any further. This is a first world book, dealing with first world problems, for first world people. I know it feels kind of egregious to talk about struggling with a sense of restlessness when people are really suffering in other parts of the world.

That phrase *first world problem* has its own hashtag on Twitter, and is a hilarious recital of superficial issues of modern life, like losing the remote when you have settled on the couch, the dog and cat are both snoring on top of you, and the blanket is tucked in nicely.

The term is a perfect description of the discontent that arises from having too much time on your hands, too much money, too much comfort, and too much opportunity to overthink things.

Yes, yes, being bored in retirement – when you have enough money to live without working and you can do whatever you like – sounds suspiciously like it qualifies as a first world problem. But wait.

I also think that it must be OK to deal with your life just as it is. You're not someone else, and what you have to deal with is to a great extent what you've been given. I do not think we should feel guilty about exploring what makes us tick. And I think Plato would agree.

"An unexamined life is not worth living", he said. So let's examine.

This book may well be a first world book, about the ennui and soul searching that come when you have nothing you *have* to do.

Think of it this way: you're at the pinnacle of Maslow's hierarchy and the need for Self-Actualization. Congratulate yourself for being at the top of the evolutionary heap.

Maybe this is what we're meant to be doing at this point in our lives. Soul searching. What a thought!

Oh I can't wait!

Before you retire you typically spend years planning and thinking about that time when you can finally do what you want – paint, write, relax in the sun, do Pilates three times a week, plant that flower garden. So you work at a job you may or may not enjoy because at some time in the future you will be able to live as you really want to live.

And maybe you plan for a move to a foreign country that offers everything you want plus the stimulation of living in a new culture.

Finally the time comes when all your finances are in place; you take a deep breath and make the plunge. You've planned for this, looked forward to it, can't wait to get started making new friends, entertaining in your new, funky place and just enjoying yourself in all your new activities.

Sound familiar? You bet. We've all been there. Looked to the future as the best time of our lives.

It's fun to begin with. Lots to do, lots of adjustments. You still can't wait until you get all this *stuff* dealt with so you can settle down and enjoy your retirement. You finally get all the details of your new life seen to and enthusiastically start joining classes, groups, and attending local cultural events. Oh the excitement!

Then…after awhile it begins to get, shall we say, a little unsatisfying? You try to ignore this but finally admit that you want something more. What? What else is there to want? Isn't it too late anyway?

No, it's not. But the truth is, retirement is an *enormous life transition* that can take you by unpleasant surprise. It's like a huge tidal wave of change sweeping over you and you may feel like you're drowning.

What the Retirement Rebel really, really wants

We Retirement Rebels want interesting things to do…but not too many. We also want a lot of free time, down time, reflective time…but not too much.

We want to feel engaged with life. We want to have something meaningful to do with our time. We also want to play and hang out with friends. Plus time to nap with the dogs.

Not a lot to ask, is it?

We want to enjoy the time we have left on this planet and be relaxed. We may not be as driven or ambitious as we used to be, but that's OK! It's time to change, it's time to reflect, and it's time to re-invent!

This book is about how to get your life to work when you retire. It's about how to avoid the blues in the first place and re-create life on your terms. The retirement blues is a modern problem—your grandpa didn't have the blues and wouldn't have a clue what we are talking about. He would be scratching his head. Your grandma would be too busy to notice.

The good news is that there are modern solutions to these modern problems. I offer them in this book; you can try them at home with no health warnings attached and you won't even need an app for them.

I'm an NLP (Neuro-linguistic Programming) life-coach and personal development trainer with over seventeen years' experience helping people make sense of their lives. I've also had my own transitions to deal with. So I'm interested in helping you through this period, in a way that enables you take full advantage of the positive aspects of growing older and not having to work anymore.

There are many. Not having to work is one. No more kids to look after on a day-to-day basis, no more cooking or cleaning (if you live in Mexico), no deadlines, no more doing things you don't like. That's got to be good, right?

Retirement can be fun and exciting and interesting. It should be the best time of your life. You've just got to be prepared for those blues so they don't blindside you.

This book is not about pensions, or savings, or insurance, or health plans. Nor will it give advice on whether to sign up for that retirement village when you still feel like a youngster. There is a wealth of information available on those sorts of issues and all of it bores me to tears. Yes, you have to take care of business, but it's so off point for me. The greatest insurance or pension scheme in the world won't take care of the blues.

What will take care of the blues is recognizing what causes them, being prepared for them and taking steps to avoid them in the first place.

That's what this book is about.

The *Four Retirement Pitfalls* that can ensnare you and how to avoid them

You, the Retirement Rebel are willing to make an effort to get it right. You don't want to waste precious time trying to figure things out and get on track. You will do what it takes to have a great life, here, now, in retirement.

This book will accelerate your transition into retirement and help you make it as smooth as possible. But you first need to know what dangers lie ahead, and what you need to look out for.

In my own journey from the doldrums to a satisfyingly smooth sailing life in Mexico, I identified the *four retirement pitfalls* that can spoil your joy and waste your time.

Here they are:

1. The pitfall of **too many changes** coming all at once, causing overwhelm

2. The pitfall of **too many choices,** causing stuck state

3. The pitfall of **too little challenge,** causing boredom and restlessness

4. The pitfall of **too much clutter,** both mental and physical, slowing you down and keeping you tied to the past.

This book will help you avoid these problems in the first place and gives great solutions to put in place to prevent them ever taking hold of you.

No more wasting precious time trying to figure out how to make retirement work for you.

So read on if you want to find out how to sail happily out of the retirement doldrums, on course, with plenty of wind in your sails, on your terms, in your control, at the speed you want, with whom you want, and enjoying every moment.

You can be the Retirement Rebel/Pirate/Reprobate/Brat— rocking retirement!

Sound good? Let's look at *Retirement Pitfall #1: Too many changes! All at once!* Watch out for this oh-so-modern problem which is common among baby-boomer-non-conformist-old-hippie-retirement rebels; it can take you by surprise and cut you adrift.

Chapter 1
Too Many Changes

"Turn and face the strange, Ch-Ch-Changes…Pretty soon now you're gonna get older" – David Bowie

A decade ago when I moved abruptly from England to Texas, I had lived in England's *green and pleasant land* for nearly thirty years.

At the same time I made this crazy move, I had just divorced, my kids were leaving home, I had to give up my career and colleagues in England, my finances were in free-fall, and I didn't look or feel good.

In the chaos I lost my identity as a sassy blonde American living in England (which was fun), my identity as a mother and business trainer (three kids, how *does* she do it?), and my identity as a wife, with the cultural security that brings.

And boy, did I not fit into Houston culture in any way, shape, or political form.

Confession time: meeting a handsome Mexican on an airplane influenced the timing of my move. I never flirt with strange men on planes but nevertheless, within six months I had packed up my company, ensured my grown up kids were settled, and flown the coop to Houston and a new life.

I thought it would be easy – after all I had grown up in Alabama, considered myself pretty adaptable and was up for an adventure in warm weather and sunshine. Oh, and a new Spanish speaking *novio* didn't hurt. What could go wrong?

Let me count the ways.

Of all people, I should have known better; as a life-coach and personal development trainer I knew full well that big life changes are best handled *ONE AT A TIME*. Let that sink in. It may save your sanity sometime. Only one life change at a time please.

Plus it's advisable to retain as much stability as possible during big transition periods in order to limit anxiety and depression. *Do it little by little* was my advice; one major change at a time. Give your psyche time to adjust before you move on to the next shock, and allow yourself recovery time.

Shame I didn't take my own counsel.

I call it *transition shock* – the anxiety and blues that can accompany times of change. I must have thought I was immune. It's hard to coach yourself.

I had created the perfect storm for major emotional challenges. The Blues. My whole life, including my roles, activities, and identity, was suddenly gone with the wind. And instead of the gentle, rolling green hills and comfy familiarity of England to ease the pain, I was in Houston.

Houston! I had landed in a flat wasteland of unbearable heat, ten lane freeways, huge pick-up trucks, and endless identical shopping malls. I felt like I had arrived in the Great American Nightmare.

I'm a softhearted animal loving, vegetarian, old-hippie-at-heart. You know, the whole bleeding heart liberal shebang. Not a good fit for Houston.

I felt like a cat with my fur standing on end. Yeah, and I come from Alabama. Go figure.

Add all this onto *a premature enforced retirement* – premature because I wasn't prepared for it and enforced because circumstances had dictated it. I no longer had my training company, and I hadn't worked at a proper job in the States or anywhere else for ages. At age fifty plus, with no work record, I wasn't eminently employable, and I didn't have the resources to restart my European training company in the States.

Hence, *premature enforced retirement.* And please don't forget the recent divorce, new partner, empty nest, loss of friends and network. Yes, the perfect storm.

Retirement Pitfall #1: Too many changes

Retirement is one of life's major transition points. It has always signified a huge disruption in lifestyle for everyone closely involved. It's an old chestnut that traditional stay-at-home wives are terrified at the prospect of newly retired husbands hanging around with nothing to do.

Simply stated, retirement is when you stop working for a living. And whether it's by choice or has been foisted upon you, it can mean big changes – in work, where you live, and in how you spend your time. It's always stressful, even when you feel happy about it.

The truth is, we hippie-at–heart baby-boomer types tend to have unsettled lives at best. Many of us no longer live with the backup of stable structures such as hometown communities, church, and close living extended families to aid us during times of change.

The role of church, family, community

As recently as forty or fifty years ago, when people retired they had traditional communities to help them cope with the turmoil that was part and parcel of retirement. They had friends they had known since childhood who were retiring at the same time. Churches provided retirement activities with other retirees. Children and grandchildren living nearby would help to take away the sense of loss or feeling old and redundant.

These days many of us live far away from our children, sometimes in different continents, and most of us do not live in the hometown where we grew up. We don't tend to participate in community or church life as much as our parents did. As a result, we have lost all that emergency support – we sacrificed it for adventure and wider horizons.

And I can't speak for you, but I wouldn't trade the life I've chosen for the safer, more secure option. I stand by my choice to be a misfit, non-conformist rebel, but boy it can be tough sometimes. It can get lonely out here in lone-wolf land.

Sanity and survival

If we want to keep our sanity during retirement, we are going to have to build our own safety structures and find new tribes we can rely on in times of stress. For this we will need freshly hewn tools to survive. We need to become Retirement Rebels.

I have three survival tools that I hewed from my own experience of transition shock.

1. The first tool is to *cocoon*.

2. The second tool is to *grieve* for what's been lost.

3. The third tool is to *find a tribe* and build new shelters to fortify against future shock.

Cocooning

Cocooning is about surrendering to the moment, with all the emotions and despair and self-doubt you may be feeling. Just let it in and stop fighting it, for now. Have that pity party and get it over with. You only get one Retirement Pity Party. Your *Oh Why Did I Retire So Early? —What Possessed Me to Move to Mexico?—Who IS This Person I'm Living With?* party. Wrap it all up in one go.

Climb in bed or on the sofa, pull up a comforter, call the dogs, grab your favorite drink, and put on your technological drug of choice. It's time to hunker down for a while.

What you're going to do is give yourself some space and time to heal and reflect. You don't need to do anything, just give yourself a break. It's OK to not be OK for a bit. I don't want you to get stuck here, but take as much time as you need.

"Oowee, are we gonna fly, Down into the easy chair!"

I find I need to cocoon after every significant change in my life, and I include travel. I get the travel blues most times I return from a big trip and I don't want to do anything or be around anyone for days. I have no idea where I am or how I got here. I frequently feel disoriented about everything in my life and go into a funk.

So I simply give myself time to readjust and sometimes I may need to take a whole week for re-entry. I do the minimum to keep alive and flip channels. Oh, I always like my dogs and cat. They are the exceptions. I remind myself that eventually I always return to normal and to just be patient with myself for however long it takes.

So cocoon for as long as you need to. Retirement is a big huge disruption and no matter how smart and adaptable and world wise you think you are, you need some space to adjust.

You will inevitably second-guess all your choices. It doesn't mean they were wrong. Every choice and decision has an equally viable opposite choice you could have made. It's OK to wonder if you chose the right one, but just hang in there, you can make this work.

Now, what you will find as you cocoon and heal is that you are missing something that is making you sad. What is it?

Grieving

Every change implies an ending to what was before.

It's normal to be blue when something is over, done, finished. It's like a death. Sometimes we can't pinpoint exactly what we are sad about – it's just an underlying feeling of unease, of *all's not right with the world.*

Retirement is a big fat ending. You are ending your work life, which you have probably been engaged in for most of your time as an adult. You've poured enormous amounts of energy into it. It is a big deal.

At first you may be in denial and unable to let go. Was retirement a bad idea? Was relocation ill advised? In the back of your mind is the thought that you might be able to go back and pick up where you left off. You maintain contact with old work colleagues. This seldom goes well. In most cases you have lost the connection that held you together and those interesting, tight friendships can vanish overnight.

We grieve for aspects of our old life, *even if we didn't like them, or are glad they are over.* You may have disliked your job, been bored with it, jaded, and even tired of the same old people. Doesn't matter. When it's gone, it leaves a hole.

You can't help but wonder if it was all a waste of time. When we stop work, it's as if it never happened. It's a weird, disconcerting feeling.

Here are some of the things you may lose when you retire: something that gets you up and dressed every day, the pressure to perform, recognition of achievements, work colleagues, a sense of where you fit in life, a sense of status. Even if you worked freelance or from home, you would have deadlines to meet and people you interacted with who had expectations of you. All that changes once you leave work.

William Bridges in his book *Transitions*, says there are two questions to ask during transition times:

1. What is it time to let go of in my life right now?

2. What is standing backstage in the wings of my life, waiting to make its entrance?

What do you need to grieve? What aspect of your work do you miss the most? It can sometimes be hidden things that you miss most deeply.

When I moved to Houston from England, what I missed most about my old job were my friends and colleagues who went through NLP (Neuro-linguistic Programming), hypnotherapy, and coach training with me. We used to meet every week to discuss our coaching clients and gather new ideas on how to handle tricky situations. We would practice our skills and techniques and just hang out and share professional experiences.

I could never, ever replace that in Houston. Although I had internet and email to keep up with old friends and I could see my kids whenever I wanted to, I could never replace that unique work situation. It was gone, over, finito, when I moved to Houston. For a long time I had no idea why I felt so unhappy whenever I thought about working again.

Once I identified the underlying problem, I was able to face it, grieve, and let it go. Eventually, I hooked up with some of those old colleagues on Facebook and that has been somewhat compensatory – but at the time of my move to Houston, Facebook was still a dream of Mark Zuckerberg. Can you remember a world without Facebook?

Make peace with your past

So, if you are feeling blue, disillusioned and unable to move forward, this is a sure sign you need to grieve for something you left behind in your old life. Try to drill down and find what it is. Sometimes bringing these lurking gremlins into the light, blinking and glaring, is all you need to do to get rid of them.

Think of it as clearing out a cupboard. You have to open it first, see what's in there and then decide what you are keeping and what you are getting rid of. Oh, I know it's not easy. I can keep closets closed for years. I will open them briefly to throw in some more junk, and then slam the door firmly for another long interlude.

If you find this a bit tough to do, simply pretend you are telling someone about your life – up to now. Or hire a coach and tell him or her. Start talking. What do you focus on? What events and achievements seem important? Who are the people in your life worth mentioning? Where did you live and what did you do?

You want and need to acknowledge your former life – celebrate it – before you let it go. Validate it, glean what you learned from it, and recognize you lived the best life you could – and let that story go. Time to write a new one.

What you resist, persists

When we resist our problems, we strengthen them.

I want to round up a sacred cow right here and bring it in for milking. Everyone from therapists to coaches to pastors and self-help gurus will tell you that you must always think positively and get rid of all negative thoughts and feelings.

Focus on the good things! They moo. Be grateful! Do not let a negative thought even enter your being. Banish it, squash it, and be positive!

Balderdash. That is impossible. A Sacred Cow indeed. Why not just relax and let all those feelings in, welcome them with a sigh and offer them a cushion in front of the fire. These negative emotions are here for a perfectly valid reason and the more you resist them, the stronger they become. So say hello and stop fighting. It's OK to feel whatever you are feeling, even if it's not especially pleasant. So what?

I encourage my clients to make lunch dates with friends and to unload and talk about their former lives. Sometimes it helps for someone to hear about your achievements and successes, to be impressed and celebrate them with you. In your new life you don't want to live in the past, but sharing it briefly with someone will help you to move on.

I did this with my coach. Having that professional perspective made me feel safe in whatever I talked about. In my new home in Mexico nobody knew who I was or what I had achieved. I didn't want to go around talking about my past, but it felt so good to let someone to know that at one time I did this, and achieved that, and got that award, and was salesman of the year way back in the Dark Ages. My coach acted suitably impressed and was then able to help me find *new* passions and *new* interests that naturally segued from the old life.

Now I'm not saying everyone has to do this. You may have a very good relationship with your past. But if you are feeling blue or melancholy, this might help.

Invite the emotions in. Sit with them. Don't resist them. Notice the story you have built up around them. Notice that the story is neither true nor false – it's just a story that keeps the emotions in place. Without the story holding it all in place, you can let the negative emotions go.

A little bit of life-coaching – give yourself permission to feel what you are feeling

Melody Beattie, in her book *Make Miracles in 40 Days,* claims that resisting sadness or grief, or any negative emotions we are having, simply reinforces them. When we repress them we go into denial.

She recommends honoring *all* emotions and writing them down every day for 40 days, preceded with the statement *"I'm grateful today for/that…"* I feel sad, or I feel down, or I'm really angry.

Don't justify or explain it, just record the emotion. It may sound counterintuitive to record negative feelings, but it's a way of acknowledging that everything that happens in our lives has meaning and ultimately fits into a larger pattern.

It's recommended to do this with a friend, sending a list to each other every day for 40 days. If you do this then make a rule that neither of you is allowed to comment on the lists. You want to avoid having to justify or explain what you have written. This gives you total freedom to express yourself.

Beattie points out that there are exceptions; for example, a tragic death or being abused. You don't say you are grateful for

25

these because that would be disrespectful and banal. However, you can acknowledge how you are feeling about it.

This is an important step in letting go. By honoring these feelings instead of fighting them, you are allowing them to release. Our unconscious mind wants us to get the lessons from our past, no matter how painful, and will cling tightly to the unpleasant emotions until we do.

Try this miracle exercise – it's remarkable. If you are feeling stuck, lost, depressed or guilty, validate these feelings. They are trying to tell you something.

Finding tribe

We old hippies/retirement rebels are tribal in spirit, but ironically tend to lack tribes. It's our choice – we didn't want to be part of the old structures of hometown and church and close-knit families. We wanted adventure and the freedom to live in exotic parts of the world and be ourselves without the constraints of societal disapproval. It was Kathmandu and Amsterdam back then – it's Bali, Costa Rica, Mexico, today. The hippies were our tribe.

"Where have all the flowers gone? Long time passing."

As mentioned earlier, many of us live far away from our children. Many of us live far away from our hometowns. Many of us live in foreign countries. Many of us live in blended families and aren't married to our first spouse. A lot of us don't belong to a spiritual or religious organization, or at least not the one we grew up with.

As a result, many of us are more or less tribe-less, and without supportive and meaningful communities we can identify with and which can help us with our transitions.

So what? Is this a problem? Well, it can be if our main tribe has been our workplace and work colleagues. Even the self-employed have workmates and clients and people they have dealings with on a regular basis.

When we retire, not only do we lose our identity connected to our work roles, we also lose our work tribe.

This matters because humans are tribal animals. We have lived in tribes since earliest times. The members of a tribe work together for survival. Each member has a role to play – and banishment from the tribe means death.

But I didn't like a lot of the people at work, I hear you cry. Or *I didn't have real friends at work.* Doesn't matter. In a tribe you don't have to like everyone. What makes a tribe a tribe is some common bond; in the work place it's the company and the job.

One of the dictionary definitions of tribe is, "Any aggregate of people united by ties of descent from a common ancestor, community of customs and traditions, adherence to the same leaders…"

So family is tribe, church is tribe, a hometown can be a tribe, a neighborhood or street can act as a tribe, and the workplace definitely provides a tribe. When we retire and move away, we may lose several tribes at once.

Being without a tribe isn't natural and it goes against archetypal human instincts. We need others and we need to be part of a group to feel safe. You need them and they need you.

Where have all our tribes gone?

Today in modern society, especially Western developed nations, the natural tribal collectives of village and family have mostly disappeared. Our cities encourage us to be disconnected from others, when our natural instincts are to connect. Our cities are lonely.

Unless we deliberately seek out tribes, we can end up isolated and alone.

Retirement exacerbates this feeling of disconnect and loneliness so it's helpful to make an effort to find new tribes that you feel connected to.

The ex-pat experience

One reason people love living in foreign countries is they feel a connection to the other ex-pats in the country. They have an automatic feeling of tribe and it's interesting and satisfying. The smaller the ex-pat community, the better the sense of belongingness.

When I moved to Mexico I remember on my first visit to the grocery store another American went out of her way to help me find what I needed. I must have looked puzzled. I had just moved from Houston and I can guarantee you I never experienced that sort of helpfulness among strangers while there. To me Houston epitomized loneliness, distrust, and mind your own business.

People who move to foreign countries report that the ex-pat experience is one of feeling *we are all in it together* and need our fellow compatriots. Giving lifts to total strangers, offering advice and directions, even putting just met friends up in your home is commonplace. Making instant friends in the park, in a restaurant, in the store, happens every day.

There is also a price to pay for membership with any tribe and that is a certain amount of conformity to spoken or unspoken rules. An ex-pat tribe usually has loose knit expectations such as: don't criticize or complain about local shortcomings, stay out of politics, and don't be arrogant. Learn the language.

Spiritual groups and churches make great tribes but tend to have tighter rules. It's important to look for ones where you feel an attraction to the beliefs propounded. You will need to buy into what they espouse because like tribes of old, non-conformity isn't easily tolerated. That's why it's important you agree with most of the creed. You're going to have to support it if you want to stay a member.

The tribal aspect is why a religion like Mormonism is so strong. Dissonance isn't tolerated, but the tribal support is powerful.

Those of us who are rebellious old hippies can have a hard time with the tribal experience. A loose knit tribe like ex-pats suits us because the rules aren't too strict. We like the social part but kick back against conformity. I probably wouldn't have survived in the Neanderthal days. I'd have been banished for being obnoxious, and eaten by wild animals

How do I find a tribe?

So what use to you now, in retirement, is this information about tribes?

Just this. You probably need one. And you do have interesting options you can choose from. We can choose and even create our tribes rather than being born into them.

You find them by putting in a bit of effort.

- To start, make sure you cultivate whatever family you have. Make an effort to ensure you meet and visit regularly. Family is automatic tribe.

- Next you might create your own group of people held together by some bond. Spiritual practice, a hobby, an interest, something. You must meet regularly for it to work. This is why churches function so well as tribes.

- Look into some sort of charity or service work. Look out for a politically active group with an agenda; this can create a powerful bond for some.

- Finally, join groups that meet regularly. Meditation groups, Buddhist groups, healing circles or whatever is of interest to you, where there are like-minded people with whom you can connect. Community work is also good, as are men's groups, women's groups, book groups, writer's circles.

Just get involved with something you enjoy and that includes people with whom you feel compatible. It takes effort, but life doesn't work so well when you are isolated.

It will pay dividends when you don't feel alone, or have to face transitions without support. Recently a single lady here in San Miguel tripped on the cobblestones and broke her knee. She had formed a tight tribe of other single ladies who shared her artistic interests. She was looked after, cooked for, had company, and her every need catered to during her entire recovery period. For free.

Questions to ponder

What groups are a natural fit for me?

What activities do I enjoy that involve other people?

With what type of people do I feel an affinity?

Homework

Grab your local newspaper or go online and find what groups meet regularly in your community.

Make a list of ones that appeal to you, or excite your interest.

Start with one, and attend a meeting. Get going and work your way through your list. There's no hurry. Give each one a chance with more than one meeting, unless there is some startling reason you don't want to go back.

Let go of expectations and just be open to whatever happens. Don't try to push friendships or connections – just let them occur naturally. Also don't judge too quickly whether there is anyone there you can connect with. If you enjoy the meeting, go again.

Things to ponder

OK! We've just looked at how too many changes all at once can affect your life and overwhelm you, especially during the big transition of retirement. The first step is to cocoon, giving yourself time and space to heal. Surrender to what is going on, allow yourself to feel whatever you are feeling, then grieve, rewrite your story and find a new tribe to help you survive.

Do this

Identify the changes you are going through in retirement.

Take each one separately and notice what emotions are involved.

Notice what you are missing, what has ended as a result of that change.

Either allow yourself to just let it go, or use one of the methods in the chapter, or failing that see a coach or therapist. Call me. No wait, use email – I've forgotten how to use the phone.

Modern Problem: too many changes going on all at once causing overwhelm, the blues, feeling disoriented. A modern phenomenon springing from our unorthodox lives and myriad choices of lifestyle. We may be going through divorce, taking up with a new partner, moving to a strange and exotic location, kids leaving home, plus retirement – happening all at the same time. *Retirement Pitfall #1.*

Old-fashioned Solution: take a break, grieve for what you have lost, talk to someone about it, and make new friends. Call home. Granny would like that.

Next, *Retirement Pitfall #2: Too many choices*! What? We slave away our whole lives in order to have more choice in life, so what in the world is this about? It makes no sense at first glance…but watch out, this pitfall will trap you and keep you imprisoned if you're not vigilant.

Chapter 2
Too Many Choices

"One is not born into the world to do everything but to do something." – Henry David Thoreau

The Hungarian psychologist Mihaly Csikszentmihalyi has been researching for many years which elements in life make us happy. Strangely, unlimited freedom of choice isn't one of those elements.

Csikszentmihalyi made the interesting observation that in the developed West we enjoy personal freedoms that would have been unthinkable a century ago and we place high value on the individual's personal freedom and right to choose.

But it's not making us happy. It seems that what we have fought so hard to achieve doesn't necessarily give us what we're after.

Let me explain… and tie this observation to retirement.

In the early twentieth century society and parents made crucial life decisions for you. Where you went to school, what career path you chose, where you lived, even whom you would marry, were pretty much dictated by circumstances. Personal freedom was the prerogative of a few brave pioneers.

Today we face a plethora of choices, opportunities, and possible roads to take on our life's journey. Even ordering a coffee comes with mind-boggling decisions. It's the Starbucks Syndrome – all you want is a cup of coffee but you are forced to choose from thirty options. Coffee with milk did you say? Latte? Cappuccino? Caramelized Honey Cappuccino? Frappuccino? Or perhaps Macchiato? Skinny Latte? Did you want it with soy or dairy? Decide please, and quickly. There are people behind you waiting in line.

Stress! Just coffee, please! This is confusing and sucks my energy. I don't want to feel stupid and slow.

It's the same in our supermarkets. You want cereal? Bread? Cat food? There are rows and rows of choices. And you really ought to read the labels to make sure the fat and proteins are balanced properly. Is it GMO free? Organic? Locally sourced?

These are great metaphors for our opportunities in life today. Overwhelming. Life used to be so simple when we had fewer choices.

Retirement Pitfall #2: Too many choices

So what? I hear you cry. Read this.

> *"The inevitable consequence of equally attractive choice is uncertainty of purpose; uncertainty, in turn, saps resolution, and lack of resolve ends up devaluing choice."*
> – *Csikszentmihalyi*

Csikszentmihalyi seems to be describing a retirement pitfall pretty well in that statement. Too much choice can confuse and exhaust rather than inspire. How to choose? What if you go for the wrong one? Ever gotten the wrong coffee? I usually do. Decision-making takes a huge amount of mental energy and we will sometimes go to great lengths to avoid it. It's called procrastination. I have been known to walk away from a drink stand because I couldn't choose what drink I wanted. Going thirsty seemed the easier option.

If you have an excess of options, *you are apt to get stuck* doing none of them. Hold on to that thought because getting stuck and doing nothing are characteristic of the blues.

Pulling your hair out

Today in boomer land when you retire you can go to any class, attend any workshop, join any group, and do and be whatever you want. Hang on, maybe I should go to India rather than Tibet. Should I start my own online business? Write a book? Volunteer in the charity bookstore? Help stray animals? Open a second hand jewelry store?

Is there something better on another channel? I need to check my email again.

When I first read what Csikszentmihalyi said about choice I jumped out of my chair and paced around the garden in excitement. It hit home like a nuclear-fired rocket. I had everything I needed – and I mean everything – to make life free, exciting, and fulfilling, and total control over how to spend my time. Yet here I was spending the afternoon reading a book and wondering what I would watch on TV in the evening.

Like an alcoholic who holds off on taking that drink until it's 5pm, I paced my TV viewing to begin at 7 and not before. That way I could pretend to have it all under control.

Finding the glue

Oh, I had plenty of activities to choose from all right. When I hit San Miguel I threw myself enthusiastically into every interesting group or class I could find. I got very busy. But after awhile it all seemed like a waste of time. Nothing seemed to relate to anything else. I felt like I needed some kind of bond or glue to make sense of it all.

Wait. That's called a job, a career, a calling, a purpose.

I had nothing compelling to do, so I ended up doing nothing. I'm the type of person who is naturally lazy so I need powerful motivators – such as the threat of imminent bankruptcy, starvation, or foreclosure on my home – to really get motoring. My new Mexican husband had enough money for us to retire comfortably in the mountains of Mexico. We can travel anywhere we like, and I can spend my time in any way that I choose. So I usually choose the couch, with dogs, iced tea, and computer.

My career and bringing up my kids had been the *glue* holding it all together in my old life. Now they were gone and with it the cohesion that gave my activities meaning and motivation. I had actually loved all the stress and challenge of work; I just needed a vacation now and then. Well, now I was on permanent vacation. Be careful what you wish for. Even TV and computer can get boring if that's all you do. (Iced tea and dogs, never.)

OK, yes I know, this is where you get the hankies out because you feel so moved by my plight. What? You don't feel sorry for me?

It calls to mind the quote from Macbeth:

"Out, out, brief candle!...It is a tale told by an idiot, full of sound and fury, signifying nothing."

That line always disturbs me. It expresses a deep-seated fear that life is a waste of time and has no meaning. Nobody wants that, but when we retire this fear seems to rear its ugly head. Was all my work life spent on a tale told by an idiot?

Surely I had something important to do, something that would use my skills and experience? I seemed to have a plethora of choices, but no ability to choose.

Caveat here: I am fully aware that having too *little* choice is equally challenging. Too little choice or too few options and we feel imprisoned and unable to break free. But I am making the assumption that for most of my baby-boomer-retirement-rebel readers this is not the case.

So what do we do with too many options?

Let's get back to Csikszentmihalyi. He seemed to have his finger on my pulse. Maybe I should read on and find if he had the solution for too much choice?

He does indeed. He goes on to say that:

- The complexity and freedom that have been thrust upon us, and that our ancestors had fought so hard to achieve, "*are a challenge we must find ways to master.*" (OK. I'm listening.)

- When there are too many demands, options, challenges, we become anxious; we burn out and then think we are bored. (Been there.)

- When we focus on what *could* be – unlimited opportunities – rather than what *is*, we become conflicted. This causes confusion. (Protestant guilt complex, please stand up. I'm never doing enough.)

- "When we can imagine only few opportunities and few possibilities, it is relatively easy to achieve harmony."

How do I do this? Imagine fewer opportunities? How does that work? Read on.

The key to harmony is to limit opportunities and possibilities

How?

Here is an example of reducing choice. At one point I thought I would try art, painting to be specific. So I joined a class…and without any doubt produced the worst work in the room. Everyone was terribly encouraging and kind, but I'm not totally unaware. My paintings were so painful to look at that people averted their eyes. (I'm kind of joking. But I won't show them to you.)

I soon came to realize that even though I quite enjoyed splashing paint on canvas, it was going to take years of slog to achieve a level of skill that would give me satisfaction. I didn't have a load of years.

So what? I hear you cry. If you enjoy it, so what? Indeed. But I wasn't getting enough positive feedback either from my own eyes or from others that what I was doing was worth the effort. We have to have feedback to keep us motivated to do anything.

I was getting feedback all right but it wasn't encouraging me. The art teacher inadvertently made it worse. *"Oh I've been working on this for forty years,"* she would chuckle. *"Give yourself a break!"* Forty years? Hello.

So I decided not to spend three or four hours a week in class working at something that I would only be OK at even after a length of time and effort. I decided instead to focus more on areas where at least I had a head start. I wouldn't feel I was wasting my time.

As human beings we are hard wired to learn, to improve, and to gain some sort of mastery somewhere. Nothing is more satisfying. (Hold on to this idea, as we will explore it in more detail later: mastery, expertise, being good at something.)

I don't regret giving up art for a moment. I tried painting and it wasn't for me. The point is, with everything you try, you are starting to limit yourself and that's a good thing.

I can always go back to it later if I want to. Look out art world. Grandma Moses may reincarnate.

Do you really want to start from scratch at this age?

So, if not art, then what was I good at?

I decided I just didn't have time or motivation to start learning something from scratch. So I began to concentrate on writing, coaching, standing in front of groups, and training. That was what I loved and what I could do with some skill. OK, so I'm not a great cook, my art is, ahem, not outstanding, and my Spanish nada. But I can do other things that not everybody can do. Why not get better at those things? That might be fun.

I cannot do everything. But I can do something. Put that on your mirror.

Retirement is the time when you can finally focus not only on what you enjoy but also on those areas where you already have some competence.

The brain fog started to clear. I started mulling over these questions.

- What skills do I already have?

- What do I enjoy doing that makes my heart sing?

- What do I have to offer the world that no one else has because they are not me?

By answering these questions you start limiting your choices. Start with throwing out things you are *not* good at, *don't* enjoy and have *no* affinity for. In other words the activities you think you *should* or *ought* or *must* do.

I confess right here that I am not cut out for charity work. I know I should do it and certainly ought to, but I have never liked it. So I work on being a decent human being in other ways.

Get rid of all the things you *should do*. See what that leaves you with. The field is narrowing. It's an exciting feeling, like being on a treasure hunt and getting closer to your prize, the Holy Grail.

My clients hammer me with this

I get these two questions all the time from my life-coaching clients here in San Miguel de Allende in Central Mexico.

- What now? What next?

- What is my life purpose?

San Miguel is a great retirement mecca for Americans and Europeans who want the year round great climate, friendly people, reasonably cheap prices, and lots of interesting stuff to do – including cooking classes, Spanish schools, art activities of all kinds, yoga events of all stripes, meditation classes, Buddhist centers, its very own Yogananda group, dancing lessons – the list goes on and on. You cannot get bored here. Or can you?

If you can't get bored then why do I have people coming to me searching for their purpose in life? What is that about? This seems to be a fairly common preoccupation among the baby boomer age group.

When I hear someone say they are looking for their life purpose I translate it as:

"I'm bored because I have too many options to choose from. Help me."

Or

"I've worked so hard to get myself to a place where I don't have to work and can pursue all those things I never had time for while I was working, and now they don't interest me much."

Phrases such as 'stuck', 'searching for my life purpose', 'trying to move to the next level', seem to be modern self-help speak for… *"I just don't know what to do with myself"*.

Finally being able to work that organic garden can be fun to start with and your first vegetables are exciting…and that's it. You eat them and they are vegetables. They may be healthy and tasty, but you can buy them for a lot less trouble at the local supermarket. It doesn't complete your life, *on its own,* unless gardening is something for which you have always had a yen and for which you've got a purpose.

Those art classes you've been dying to try…you're sure you'll get around to signing up for one eventually. When you do join, well, it doesn't satisfy *on its own,* unless you've always had a yearning for art.

That spiritual group you finally got yourself up and dressed to go to was lovely for the first four meetings, then started to become repetitive and some of the people annoyed you.

The Spanish classes you were so looking forward to make you bleed from the ears.

Pilates? Yoga? Great. Next?

Ah, charity work! Service! That surely will be fulfilling and give meaning to life. But you can't stop second-guessing the value of what you are doing, and you really don't enjoy it as much as you thought you would...unless you're a true activist or caretaker.

Now don't get me wrong. There is absolutely nothing wrong with any of these pastimes. But what you may find is that on their own and without an underlying life theme, they can feel pointless. There needs to be coherence for them to be satisfying.

What do I mean by coherence?

Hmm, I'm feeling a new age dictum coming on – maybe you need to *find your life purpose* to get all this frantic activity to mean something? To hold it all together?

Let's get something clear first. I don't believe we have *one* life purpose. I think we have purposes for different times in our lives. So we can have more than one.

What you deemed your life purpose when you had a career will almost certainly not fit the bill when you are retired. Ah, but once again, what do we choose instead for our new life? So many options!

Choosing a life purpose can be overwhelming

I've been obsessed with finding my life purpose – a burning obsession and reason for living – for years now. It fascinates me. The implications are enormous. (Who says we are here for a purpose? Who decides what it is?)

After reading every book available on the subject and listening to countless webinars and seminars, my result was a huge amount of stress and frustration that simply increased the more I agonized over finding this elusive unicorn. Life purpose needs to be something big, grand, or something that will leave a legacy. Right? I couldn't for the life of me think what would fit that bill.

Books and websites and trainers and self-help gurus proclaim the importance of finding your one true life purpose. Without it, they breathe, you are a lost soul, wandering in the desert; your life meaningless, frustrated, and bereft of value.

I recently read about someone admitting to spending over $50,000 on one expensive life-coach to discover her life purpose. And the answer she found? She was *'meant to inspire'*. Well shoot. I could have fed her that bromide for one-tenth the price.

We are simply inundated with choices about life purpose. Who in the world could choose from so many options, especially when *meant to inspire* is one of them?

My grouch is simply this, that insisting people must find their *one life* purpose in order to be complete – their unique burning passion in life – frequently causes unhappiness, not fulfillment. It's just overwhelming. Not to mention hard on the wallet.

And I'm beginning to think this, that the sooner we lay this turkey to rest, the better for our stress levels and peace of mind.

Isn't the real desire lurking beneath the search for life purpose to find *something to do* with your time that feels productive, useful, meaningful, and absorbing? Right now? Read those last two words again – right now. That means at this time of your life.

Life purpose or 'theme'?

I prefer the word 'theme' instead of purpose. I'll tell you why. It's friendlier. Purpose is grand and spiritual and pompous sounding.

Theme is 'a unifying or dominant idea, motif, etc., as in a work of art'. I like that. It's not scary.

Instead of looking for purpose, figure out your theme in life right now. What are you about? What do you stand for? What makes your heart sing?

If you had to describe yourself and who you were and what you were all about in thirty seconds, what would you say? You know, the classic elevator speech about you?

You can no longer identify with your work, so what's your new story?

Let's narrow it down – service or healing?

The search for purpose is a search to find something worthwhile to do, something that gives meaning to your existence. And if it's not about making money it's about making the world a better place. Making a difference.

When you retire you no longer have to work to survive and you are no longer bringing up your family. Those were your themes before. Now life has changed. It's time to give back – the natural, archetypal order of things. When you are young you gather, collect, make money, provide. When you no longer have to do that, you stop taking and start giving.

I believe we have two options when we retire: service or healing. Oh yes, there is the third, doing nothing. In which case it's

45

"a tale told by an idiot, full of sound and fury". You don't want that. I know because otherwise you wouldn't be reading this book.

Service is giving back and contributing at a public level. It can be charity work, starting a dog rescue center, getting involved politically, becoming active in saving the environment; anything active, socially involved, that makes the world a better place.

Healing is helping at the personal level. It can involve physical, emotional, or spiritual healing of any kind, such as energy healing, massage, chiropractic, teaching yoga, or coaching, therapy, hypnotherapy, mentoring, meditation. Healing is for the individual.

Of course, service is healing, and healing is service, and you can contribute at both the social and personal level. They are two sides of the same coin – giving back. Making the distinction simply helps you choose which mode you will use.

Ponder these questions:

- What skills do you have?

- What do you enjoy doing?

- What are you good at?

- What have you learned from the work you've done over the years that is worth using?

- Do you prefer working with groups at the public level or with individuals?

Notice if any ideas are taking shape. You want something that excites you, makes your heart sing.

Now take the next step:

- What have you got to offer the world that nobody else has?

- What challenges have you overcome that you could help others with?

- What are you uniquely designed and prepared to do?

These were the questions that really hit home for me. Sometimes we can fall into the trap of believing we have nothing to offer that will make a difference. So stop and ponder this – there is nobody else who has your unique combination of experience, challenges and skills. Nobody. So each one of us has something we can offer the world that nobody else can.

Final question:

You have identified whether you want to be a service person or a healing person. You have your unique skill set and experiences in mind. Now how is this going to manifest in the world?

- What is the best way to deliver your service or healing?

Do you want to start a charity using your management skills? Do you want to open a wildlife rescue center using your vet skills and love of animals? Do you want to work with orphans using your caretaker skills combined with your love of children? An art gallery? A yoga center? Become a Reiki healer? Learn massage and set up a practice? Write books?

For me, it was restarting my coaching practice, and running workshops. Then later writing self-help books for people who have experienced similar challenges, like you.

Here is some extra help from an unexpected source. Hang on for the ride. This will be fun.

Archetypes do the choosing for you

When I moved to Houston and was desperately casting about to find a new direction, I picked up a book in the bookstore (remember them?) entitled *Sacred Contracts* by Caroline Myss. It was all about archetypes and she describes how each of us has a unique set that forms personality and character.

I clearly recall a light bulb exploding in my skull when I got home and started reading the book. It was as if I had discovered the lost secrets of the universe or the Philosopher's Stone. I had a burst of recognition and knowing that actually got me up off the sofa.

"Archetypes are universal forms of cosmic intelligence," Myss says. Say again?

"They are part of a person's spiritual chronology and are so ancient they predate our physical birth. Our archetypal inheritance is prehistoric, primal."

Hmm, still not clear? Keep going. You'll get it.

Carl Jung, the well-known Swiss psychiatrist and psychotherapist, was the first to use the term Archetype to signify *ancient patterns of personality* that appear in the world's myths, legends, and folk tales. They are they characters you play in your life's story, the essence of different personality types, the prototypes of different styles of character.

This is metaphorical language, so it's allowed to be a bit obtuse...but we're getting there. Or somewhere.

What makes your heart sing? Archetypes will zero in and explain it all

We seem to be born with our archetypes already in place, and they dictate what kind of person we are, what we like to do, and what we are good at. Doesn't your mother say you were always X from the word go or that you always loved doing X?

My mother says I came into the world furious and fighting. Typical Aries. A *Natural Brat*.

I have a very dominant *Seeker* archetype, which means I love to read and study and trawl for new ideas and knowledge. Nothing excites me more than learning something new…like when I discovered archetypes.

The *Seeker* dictates what I crave doing most, and also what drives my behavior and life choices. I'm always up for the next workshop, book, online course, and am always seeking fresh insights and wisdom. I can drive those around me crazy – *What? Another guru/ religion/exercise/diet/pilgrimage/seminar? What about the last one?*

Next!

I also have the *Rebel/Old Hippie at Heart*, *Adventuress* and the *Pioneer* archetypes. The *Pioneer* is related to the *Seeker*; I feel compelled to explore and be at the cutting edge and get bored if something becomes too popular or mainstream.

What's new?

The *Adventuress/Flirt* encouraged me to give my phone number to a complete stranger on an airplane to London. We've been married eight years now.

She's been retired now to keep me out of trouble.

My *Rebel* makes me question the status quo and push back against being told what to do or think. It encourages me to be honest and true to myself, and can also make me annoying and contrary. I blame being obnoxious on my *Rebel*.

I don't agree with that statement.

I have a *Teacher/Coach* archetype and love to share what I've learned with others, whether they like it or not. In fact, this archetype figured closely in helping me choose a new path in teaching and leading seminars.

In my experience...

Do you get the idea? You have your own family of archetypes, almost certainly different from mine. Take a look at this limited list (archetypes are infinite in number) and see which ones resonate with you.

Activist, Artist, Athlete, Business person, Caregiver, Magical Child, Coach, Damsel in Distress, Dilettante/Dabbler, Empath, Engineer, Organizer, Shaman, Free Spirit/Old Hippie, Healer, King/Queen, Prince/Princess, Lover (including animals, nature), Mystic, Networker, Pioneer, Pirate, Poet, High Priest/Priestess, Rebel, Rescuer, Seeker, Scientist, Student, Teacher, Warrior, Witch.

If you want a more complete list, plus clear descriptions of each archetype, go to Myss' book *Sacred Contracts*, or alternatively to the list at the back of my book *Rebellious Aging: A Self-help Guide for the Old Hippie at Heart*, both available on Amazon.

How do Archetypes relate to retirement?

Archetypes help you understand who you are and why you behave as you do: your archetypes help you figure out what will bring most joy and fulfillment in this next phase of life. They make decisions for you. Limit your choices.

My *Seeker* explains why I will default to reading if nothing else is compelling – I love exploring new ideas. My sister on the other hand has an *Athlete* archetype and she will default to playing tennis at any opportunity.

If you have an *Artist* archetype, you will be happiest pursing artistic endeavors. If an *Engineer* you may always be inventing something new. You just can't help yourself.

Archetypes help you figure out how to live appropriately for this time of life.

- Which archetypes resonate with you?

- Which archetypes seem to express your personality?

- What messages do they have for you?

- Which archetypes can help you find what you need to be doing right now?

- Which archetypes have been neglected and need to be honored?

Pulling it all together

Ponder these questions. Get to know your archetypes and they will happily take over and run your life for you.

Imagine that all your life experiences were chosen deliberately by your archetypes before you were born in order to develop and hone you for some task. What have they trained you for?

- How can you combine your archetypes, your natural propensities, and the skills you've acquired over the years? To what direction does it point?

So…

Modern Problem: having too many choices in life. Another modern 'problem' that we ironically have worked so hard to create. But with all our freedom, education, wealth, and independence we actually end up doing little more than sitting on our computers all day. *Retirement Pitfall #2.*

Old-fashioned Solution: start winnowing; ditch outdated notions of what you should or ought to be doing, and combine with what you are good at and enjoy. The result will be your true heart's desire. Do you recall what your mother said you always enjoyed doing? Check it out.

Find a way to serve that makes you happy. Get busy helping others so you don't have time to be blue.

Let's move on to *Retirement Pitfall #3: Too little challenge.* Definitely this is a modern issue. We are healthy, wealthy, and comfortable in a way our ancestors couldn't have even dreamed.

Is this a problem? Yes it is. Without challenge we get fat, soft and lazy. Today, modern Arab kings, descended from desert dwelling royalty, recognize this problem. Every year they go out to the desert and live in tents for several months, riding camels, sleeping under the stars, no cell phones in sight and sans air-conditioning, ice, and all the other comforts of modern living. They believe it keeps them hard and strong.

This is a tough one for someone who doesn't like to do anything just for the sake of it. If I can lie on the couch, that's what I'll choose. Oh please, not the tents...

Chapter 3
Too Little
Challenge

"You grow old when you lose interest in life, when you cease to dream, to hunger after new truths and to search for new worlds to conquer. When your mind is open to new ideas, new interests, and when you raise the curtain and let in the sunshine and inspiration of new truths of life and the universe, you will be young and vital." – Joseph Murphy

Mihaly Csikszentmihalyi, discussed in the previous chapter, is also known as the architect of the modern psychological concept of *flow* – a state of being totally absorbed in an activity.

His initial research unearthed the conundrum that people are not especially happy at the very times they expect to be, for example when retired and able do whatever they want, or on vacation and able to relax completely from hectic lives.

In fact, what unfolded was that provided they had effective ways to deal with stress, their *hectic* lives – their work and careers – were providing them satisfaction and happiness, but it just wasn't recognized.

In other words, the very activities that people expect to bring happiness frequently do just the opposite. That vacation became a snooze fest when it went on too long, and retirement? Forget it, tedious and empty after the initial relaxation and readjustment period was over.

So what does make us happy? Is it a human tendency to always want what we don't have and take for granted what we do have? Is the grass always greener on the other side of the fence…or can we learn to enjoy the grass in our own yard?

According to Csikszentmihalyi, there is indeed quite a lot we can do about it. We can in fact *create* happiness if we follow a few rules.

Hang in there with me. It's really quite an eye opener. These concepts have affected my choice of activities enormously and changed my life for the better. If I am stuck in the doldrums, they never fail to get me sailing again.

Csikszentmihalyi identified what was missing in our lives when we are unhappy or feeling discontented – a state of enjoyment he calls *flow* – and his contention is that human beings are happiest when they achieve *flow*.

What is *flow*?

You are in *flow* when you are engaged in an activity that is *challenging* and for which you have some skill. Where challenge and skill intersect, you lose yourself: time and ego disappear. You become totally absorbed and blissfully concentrated on the task at hand.

Flow is not the same as relaxation or even ecstasy though it does create bliss. It must have the element of challenge to qualify as *flow*. Lying on the beach is not *flow*. Having a massage is not *flow*. Sorry, sex is not *flow*. These activities are enjoyable and relaxing, but ultimately short-lived and not the panacea for discontent.

They don't fulfill the criteria for *flow*, which is what makes us deeply and sustainably happy.

Flow needs to include these six criteria:

1. The activity is challenging and you possess relevant skills for it

2. You become completely absorbed, concentrated, focused

3. You have clear goals and get immediate feedback

4. You have a sense of control

5. During the activity you forget yourself

6. There is a sense of timelessness

Retirement Pitfall #3: Too little challenge

Now let's look more closely at this. *Flow* is when challenge meets skill level. In other words, my competence is up to a challenging task. Oh that feels good! I can do something, but it isn't easy, *so it has value for me* and gives me a feeling of accomplishment. Can you remember that feeling when you've been working hard at something and you finally get it right? You're so empowered you could conquer the world.

However, if something I'm trying to do is too challenging, and my skill is not quite up to it, I get stressed or anxious. Overwhelmed. If it's too easy, I get bored.

Painting a picture, writing, making music, sports, cooking, or public speaking can put you in *flow*.

Artists, musicians and athletes are all familiar with the *flow* state. I'm sure you are too. When you are in *flow* the unconscious mind takes over and rational thinking stops. You become unconsciously competent. It's the sweet spot, when you peak. In the zone.

You are in *flow* anytime you totally forget yourself, lose your sense of time, the adrenaline is flowing, and you have enough energy to do the important task at hand. In addition there is a sense of pride inherent in being able to accomplish the task, and it fits into the overall context of your life.

My friends who love to go out dancing say their feet don't hurt and their backs don't ache…until they get home. They totally forget themselves; the dancing serves several purposes such as good exercise and social interaction. They have trained for it, taken lessons, and practiced. They feel expressive, creative, and unself-conscious – in other words, in *flow*.

It's not just physical experiences that can create *flow*. You can get into *flow* while

- Reading – if there is a purpose to it

- Socializing – if the conversation is expressive and stimulating

- Playing chess – not everyone can play this, so it has value, and you need to focus intently

- Playing games – some knowledge and skill required

- Crosswords – they challenge your literacy

- Art appreciation – if you have some art education

- Listening to music – if you have musical knowledge.

The precise balance between skill and challenge results in pure pleasure.

Flow can be addictive and this could explain certain patterns of strange behavior we observe in people. Wonder what's going on with that self-made millionaire who blew his whole fortune and had to start again? Sometimes several times? Maybe it's because the challenge of having to pick up the pieces and rise again from the ashes *puts him in flow* and that's when he feels really alive. Sounds crazy, but we really do crave feeling obsessed with what we are doing. It's a total buzz to work really hard to achieve something when there is a lot at stake.

Remember at the end of the compulsive television series *Breaking Bad* (spoiler alert!), when the lead character confesses to his wife his real reason for getting involved in the drug world? She snaps, *"Don't tell me again it was for the family!"* He says no. It was because it made him feel totally alive. When he was tangled up in the tortuous, dangerous web he had spun he was totally in *flow* and felt competent and badass. His home-cooked drugs were renowned in the underworld and he discovered capabilities he never dreamed he possessed. What made him feel alive killed him, but he died with no regrets. A perfect tale of the addictive power of *flow*.

You know people who move from relationship to relationship. Why? Perhaps starting a new relationship is a challenge that puts them in *flow*. Maybe they excel at that beginning bit where you have to be on your toes and behaving well. It gets boring once the prey is snagged.

Other people move location a lot. Same reason applies. The adrenaline fix of starting anew puts them in *flow*.

There is a lot of evidence that we take inexplicable action, get involved in dangerous sports, jump from airplanes, take drugs (a fake flow), get involved in illegal activities, and all kinds of risky stupid business so that we can experience *flow*. Gamblers love the feeling of *flow* when they are gambling. The adrenaline pumps and they feel real, alive, on the edge.

Fortunately there are plenty of safer and tamer activities that will get us in *flow* without risking home and health. We're going to find them. They are just as enjoyable as any bungee jump.

So what's the deal with retirement?

"Although, as we have seen, people generally long to leave their places of work and get home, ready to put their hard-earned free time to good use, all too often they have no idea what to do there." – Csikszentmihalyi

Csikszentmihalyi found that work – paid work – where we are held accountable for our performances provides the most readily available resource for flow and fulfillment. Ironically many push back against work, and can't wait to leave. Some think of it as an imposition, a constraint and an infringement on freedom, and therefore something to be avoided as much as possible. They crave holidays, vacations, days off, and long to retire and leave it all behind.

But assuming the work is suitable, it provides ready-made challenges along with immediate feedback, and requires skill to accomplish what is asked of you.

Think about it – what is missing when you give up work? Challenge! No more opportunity to use your hard earned skills gleaned from a lifetime of learning to achieve something that has value and meaning and recognition.

We talked about boredom earlier. Boredom comes from not having enough challenge in our lives. Full stop. Sounds kind of like retirement for a lot of people.

Purpose and flow are related

Discover and remind yourself what causes you to be in *flow*. Recall times when you were totally fulfilled with what you were doing, so much so that you felt it was what you were put on earth to do. You were excited, challenged, and happy. This will be where your true heart's desire lies. If you want to have passion and juice and purpose in your life you must first ascertain what puts you in *flow*.

Using the six criteria (repeated below) you can start to assess what you are doing in your life and if it is in line with a purpose.

You can start to pinpoint why certain activities leave you unsatisfied, and what you can do to rectify them.

Use this as a checklist for everything you do:

1. The activity is challenging and you possess relevant skills for it

2. You become completely absorbed, concentrated, focused

3. You have clear goals and get immediate feedback

4. You have a sense of control

5. During the activity you forget yourself

6. There is a sense of timelessness

For example, learning Spanish overwhelms and bores me at the same time (not a good combo), and I just switch off. If I put this through the *flow* criteria I can see that I'm not getting enough feedback that my Spanish study is being effective. The feedback I get actually tells me the opposite: that I'm wasting my time studying the subjunctive and that I will never, ever in this lifetime understand a conversation held between Mexicans. I have lots of proof to back this up.

Clearly I need a method of learning that gives me a chance to feel I'm mastering each section as I go along. Then I would gain a sense of control and enjoyment. I'm still working on it. I wonder what would happen if more teachers knew about *flow* and how important a sense of mastery, of making progress is to the learning experience.

Questions to play with

Finding flow:

- When have you been in flow?

- What activities cause you to be in flow?

- What activity totally absorbs you?

- When have you been so totally immersed in something that you forgot to eat or drink or rest? And, you felt high as a kite afterwards?

Explore all these questions. Some of them may resonate, and I suspect at least one of them will hold the key to your true longings and desires.

Write down your answers.

What patterns do you see?

What do these answers point to as your true heart's desire? Your purpose?

Conclusion

Modern Problem: too little challenge. In this chapter we have looked at the consequences of not having enough challenge in life and how it affects us in retirement. *Retirement Pitfall #3*.

When we retire we lose our major source of *flow*, so if we want to enjoy life we need to replace the *workflow* with new sources of challenge.

Old-Fashioned Solution: get busy and stop being lazy. It won't make you happy to lie on the couch all day. You have to trust me on this. You may want to explore which activities put you in *flow* and then ensure you incorporate them into your life. Finding *flow* is the best way to combat the blues.

NOTHING will make you happier than overcoming a challenge and getting lost in that challenge. Read that again. Nothing.

It may be difficult to make an effort when you don't have to. But this is one time I advise using willpower to get started. It's well worth the effort and will bring joy back into your life. That's a promise.

On to *Retirement Pitfall #4: Too much clutter.* Is this a modern phenomenon? Yes, because we are talking about mental clutter from too much technology. We also talk about physical clutter, but the mental and emotional stuff is far more intrusive.

This is a rogue wave that will leave you dead in the water, so be careful.

Chapter 4
Too Much Clutter

"You do not need to leave your room. Remain sitting at your table and listen. Do not even listen, simply wait, be quiet, still and solitary. The world will freely offer itself to you to be unmasked, it has no choice, it will roll in ecstasy at your feet." – Franz Kafka

Hmm. *"...be quiet, still and solitary"*. How many of us do that very often? It seems as if we frantically try and do the opposite, stuffing our minds and spirits with as much information as we can. Many put on the computer first thing in the morning with that first cup of coffee. Then the radio or TV while eating, and during the day something is usually going on in the background – talk shows or news – and smartphones, iPods, laptops are seldom out of reach from dawn till dusk. Netflix, videos, YouTube put us to sleep.

We are saturated with news and mind junk from various sources all day long. Do you think we might be overdoing the technological input? Just a bit?

Do you think it might be affecting our mood? Just a lot?

Chances are, like most of us, you are suffering from too much input, too much stimulation, too much information. This addiction to input will overheat your poor brain and over stimulate your emotions, suck your energy, and leave you exhausted and depressed.

Retirement Pitfall #4: Too much clutter – mental, emotional, and physical

Problem is, when we retire we have all this time on our hands and too little to do. The temptation to fill that time with technological input is strong.

Think I'm overstating? Think again. How much time are you spending during the day with something techie going on? Research reports retired people are spending up to four hours a day *on television alone!* That doesn't include internet. How much time is being spent on the internet? Radio? Phone? Looking at newspapers? Reading magazines? The opportunities for stimulation are legion. Most of us shift from one to the other so that something is always feeding our overexcited, over stuffed brains.

You can almost always trace a blue mood back to something you read or saw on the news. News is dedicated to making you angry, afraid, or sad.

Then there's gossip. Gossip is there to titillate, forcing you to judge people you don't know, and feel outraged about their behavior. Decide what you think about this person! Tweet your opinion! Notice that everything you read on the internet or news evokes an emotional reaction – which one is it? Start paying attention. *Ah, that one on the latest horrible African disease is trying to make me afraid.* Reporting always has an agenda and that's to get your attention. Emotions are click-bait.

As a result we let people we don't even know pull our strings and dictate our moods.

None of this puts us in flow. Flow activities energize us, technology drains us.

Confession time here: I find all of this extremely bothersome. My default mode is to have my little MacBook Air (upon which I am typing this very moment) either glued to my lap, or at least within reach, and always fully charged. I go from that to reading something on my Kindle and I use my iPhone to play music in the car. I listen to YouTube when cooking or tidying and in the evening I binge on Netflix. I take my computer to bed with me for more stimulating and disturbing bedtime stories.

So feel good. No matter how bad you think you are I bet it isn't as bad as I am. Or was. Or can be if I let down my guard and get lazy. It would be difficult.

And I am aware that it's not doing me any favors. At times it feels like my brain is overcooking. It needs to cool down, relax, and lie fallow for a while. I need to put it in the fridge or a bucket of ice water.

Ever notice how when you turn the noise off, it feels so blissful?

Just because you don't take drugs doesn't mean you don't have an addiction

We just don't like calling ourselves addicts. But we are. We are addicted to mental stimulation.

Addictions will happily monopolize your time for you. They take away your need to make decisions and choices, and anesthetize your worry and frustration. Addictions control time.

The definition of addiction is when the questionable behavior impinges on your quality of life. You are willing to lose the respect of others to engage in it, you take risks for it, you forgo social courtesies for it, and you make excuses for it. You defend it desperately. It's called denial.

I would call using your phone at the table in a restaurant while in the company of others, or pretending you are not wasting time but doing something useful when you've been on the computer for four hours, looking at your phone when walking your dog or taking your kids to the playground, texting while driving – all that indicates addiction to me.

Yes, you know what I'm talking about; pick your time-wasting drug of choice. And don't tell me it's not possible to spend whole days on the computer, checking email, Facebook, Huff Post, YouTube, or other online news. Maybe not lethal, but a huge time sink nevertheless.

We are worried that time is running out, so we waste it. Go figure.

Now I'm assuming that you are like I am in this respect. I'm an old hippie so discipline isn't my strong point. I do know people for whom this is not a problem. They can discipline themselves to do what they want to do and get lots accomplished without any external pressure. Bless their socks. I have to work hard at it.

Time for a brain cleanse?

Wouldn't it feel good to lose some of that stuff you're carrying around in your head all the time? You'd be amazed what happens when you do. *But what would I do with myself without my computer?* you ask. Indeed, I have said that to myself many times. What would I do if I couldn't read or listen to stuff on YouTube?

Probably feel quite peaceful.

Smoking relaxes me, says every addict. *A drink makes me more sociable,* says the alcoholic. Addicts can be wonderfully inventive with excuses. You are in denial if you say that the computer keeps you in touch with the world and oh yes, social media keeps you in touch with your friends. Sure, true, and that takes more than twenty minutes a day? I wrote the book on excuses, plus I'm a life-coach and hypnotherapist. I've heard them all before and use them myself. It won't wash.

The other evening the electricity blew out while I was home alone watching TV. I panicked for a moment as I couldn't access internet and the candles weren't bright enough for reading. My husband was out of town so I couldn't even have a conversation. Ah wait, my Kindle! Salvation! Thank goodness it was charged up! I went to bed early and read for hours. It was fun! I had little choice about how to spend my time so I just relaxed into it.

Eventually the lights came back on and I was almost disappointed. I had enjoyed the lack of options. I had been able to focus.

In the pre-electricity days, people must have done something in the evenings.

Try this

Just start doing some things without technological input. I'm not suggesting you go cold turkey because you do need your technology for some useful things – unlike alcohol, smoking, or sugar for instance. You can banish smoking or sugar or alcohol completely from your life with no ill effects. But I concede the computer has uses.

And like Eckhart Tolle says, you don't need to be violent with yourself. If you must watch TV, then at least mute it during the ads, and get up and walk around a bit. No need to swear off all entertainment just because you are prone to overdo it!

Instead of your addiction activity, do some of these. Not all the time, just some of the time.

- Take a walk with the dog without your phone, or at least don't use it.

- Cook your dinner without listening to anything.

- Sit in the garden without music or your computer nearby.

- Clean the house without entertainment to distract you in the background.

- Clean your kitchen in five minute breaks during the TV ads.

- Try driving without the radio or music on.

- When someone is talking to you, close down your computer and put your phone away.

- Take ten minutes out of your day to meditate. Sit by a tree. Listen to the birds. Do nothing and the universe will roll at your feet.

- Imagine you are just draining all the junk out of your brain.

- Put your phone away when you are in a restaurant with others at your table.

- When you get home after an afternoon out, at least take off your coat before you hit the computer.

- Use a kitchen timer when on the computer and when it rings, get up, go outside, take a breath, and do some exercise before you get back to the beast.

- Do not answer your phone or look at messages while a warm, living human being is sitting in front of you. Ever. It's not OK.

Whatever that other person on Facebook or email or Twitter wants is not more important than the person in your presence. There are VERY few instances of emergency when you must answer your phone. What? You need to give an answer to an offer on your house? Someone is sick and you need to hear from him? How often does this happen? If you do have an urgent genuine need to use your phone, explain to the people around you beforehand. It is just common courtesy.

I went to Tibet a few years back and was unable to access internet for weeks at a time. I was disconcerted to find how little I had missed when I finally hit an internet café and eagerly logged into civilization from the top of the world. Not much of interest. I made sure everyone was still alive and no disasters had struck and that was it. I guess I live a boring life.

When I got back home it took me a while to get back in the swing of social media. I had to work at it to get interested again! Does that tell you something? That it's really not important enough to warrant so much of our time?

I promise, the stuff will still be waiting for you when you finish your conversation or meal or meditation. You can fill up your brain again, but it's highly beneficial to empty it now and then. Give it a break.

A big cause of stress

As human beings we are not evolved to deal with non-stop news and information. Maybe in the future we will be. But for now we are only adapted to deal with what is going on around us in our immediate environment. Not much more. The next village is nothing to do with you. Your nervous system simply cannot cope with all the cruelty, death, and other awful things going on in far away parts of the world. It causes emotional overload and huge amounts of unnecessary worry and pain.

The stress comes from not being able to do one blessed thing about it. Most of it is totally out of your hands.

Stress, in turn, can cause health issues, lack of motivation and burnout. Not good. The Blues!

But here's the secret. It's the feeling of being out of control that does the most damage.

Think about it. When we move house and things don't go as planned (ever!), or we retire and find we're not having any fun, maybe we lose money on an investment, or our spouse tells us out of the blue they are leaving for a younger model – yikes! We feel insecure, threatened, and afraid of what the future holds for us. We no longer feel we are in the driver's seat and life seems to be spinning out of control.

When you hear news about terrorist attacks on the other side of the world, or some Neanderthal dentist killing a beautiful lion, or the destruction of nature, or a nightclub shoot-up, it's that helpless feeling that causes so much distress. What can I do?

The good news is there are three questions you can ask in any situation in order to begin to regain control and get your equilibrium back:

1. Can I do anything about it?

2. Can I come to terms with it?

3. Can I walk away from it?

One of these has to be a *yes*, otherwise something has to give and you don't want it to be your sanity. Let's look more closely:

1. *Can I do anything about it?* If you can do something about the situation, then take action. Just do it. Stress dissolves in relation to action taken.

2. *Can I come to terms with it?* If you really cannot change it, can you learn to accept it, live with it, or resign yourself to it – just let it go?

3. *Can I walk away from it?* If it's a no to both of the first two questions then the third option is – can you simply *get the hell out of Dodge?* Break off that relationship, move back home, or find another job. You know that romance is never going to work. You know you'll never be happy living in Kansas. Call the realtor. Turn off the news.

These are your choices. Eckhart Tolle says of course we have one more choice – to suffer. That may not be one you want to choose unless you enjoy suffering. I doubt that's you. So catch hold of one of the other three and try it out. These questions are amazing. You can pay a lot of money to get advice this effective.

Grab those reins and get back in the saddle.

Worry

Another very good reason you want to reduce all this input and mental clutter is because it creates fear for the future. We call this worry. That's when you imagine things that could happen, that might happen, but that haven't yet. You keep reading that the world as you know it is imminently close to collapse. Worse, that your investments are in danger, even more worse you will get cancer for sure. If not that, then you will die in a terrorist attack, get Zika virus, or Ebola. It used to be AIDS, remember?

Can you do anything about it? Yes, sometimes. Then take prudent action and forget about it.

No? Then forget about it. Push the delete button. It's OK. Give yourself permission to stop worrying about things that haven't happened yet.

We all have to deal with stuff when it happens to us. People will die. Money will disappear. Health issues will arise. Your loved ones will cope. You will cope. Or you won't. There's no point in coping or not coping with events ahead of time and being unhappy. Deal with them in their own appointed time, not before.

Habits – friend or foe?

Too much stimulation is a habit. Are habits invariably good or bad?

Habits have helped us to use our brains and evolve into these problem solving and creative beings that we are – residing at the top of the food chain.

Our subconscious, reptilian brains are enormously protective of habits. They like us to have habits. So when you try and mess with a habit you are coming up against primordial forces that will resist you to the death if they have to.

Why and how do we form habits?

The reasons are kind of intriguing.

A habit is an unconscious behavior and there is an evolutionary purpose behind it. We are hardwired to create habits: our subconscious mind will immediately make a behavior automatic when we do it several times. One reason is to free up brain space for more important work.

Without habitual behavior our brains would have to become huge in order to accommodate all the thinking cells required for day-to-day activity. Our skulls would need to be huge and we couldn't give birth anymore to such large headed babies. We would die off as a species.

Brain space is the most valuable bit of real estate on the planet. The more behaviors that become habitual, the more brain cells we can utilize for more important subjects. Makes evolutionary sense.

In fact, most day-to-day behaviors become automatic after some repetition. So you can drive your car, a complicated activity, while rehearsing your speech to the board of directors. You can brush your teeth while designing a rocket engine. Automatic behavior is very useful.

However, some habits don't serve you as well as others. And when you try to change them, trust me, the mind will inevitably provide obstacles to stop you. It's called self-sabotage.

Nothing can seem harder to change than a habit – even seemingly harmless habits that don't involve physical addiction. Try tweaking *any* habitual behavior and you will suddenly find yourself up against pre-historic forces so deeply ingrained and hard to shift it will make your eyes water.

Try not logging on for a full day. A half-day. OK, for a few hours. Think it's not a habit? That's a nice way to put it.

The Saboteur

The Saboteur is that part of your deep subconscious mind that will resist any and all change, just because it finds change threatening. Change is danger. Deep down the Saboteur really is your friend and protector, but it doesn't always play that way.

Attempting to use willpower alone against this powerful nemesis will probably not work and be a huge waste of energy.

The Saboteur *can* be persuaded to help you if you convince it that changing a habit is in your best interests. If it's in the organism's best interests, then it's in the Saboteur's best interests. You need to convince it of this and suggest a new habit that is more useful. But you have to be clever and subtle.

Check out this great technique. It's so simple and yet so effective. It's the main one I use to *counter* bad habits and it works really well for me – and I have a very strong and active Saboteur. I can trick it sometimes. It's not all that smart, just stubborn.

Countering technique

Countering is a technique for handling problem behavior, explicated in the book *Changeology* by John Norcross. Countering is simply substituting a more useful behavior for one you don't like. According to Norcross it is *"simple in principle: do the healthy opposite of the problem behavior."*

The idea is that two opposite behaviors cannot exist at the same time, so you are driving out the old behavior by substituting it for the new one.

So you start by asking: what is the healthy opposite or alternative to my problem?

Countering is a way of dealing with a bad habit, or a non life-threatening addiction. This is a gentle, easy and effortless way to change something that isn't working for you, but nevertheless you find compulsive and can't seem to alter no matter how hard you try.

Countering involves *accepting* rather than *fighting* the unwanted behavior. Instead of struggling with it, you simply begin replacing it, or countering it, with more desirable behaviors. For instance, if you spend too much time on the internet for your liking, you can begin replacing that habit with taking a walk, writing, doing art, or any behavior you'd prefer.

Countering works because you are being gentle with yourself. You are not beating yourself up, but nevertheless have a firm plan for replacing undesirable activities.

The Saboteur is lulled into complacency because it doesn't realize you are making changes. Fight it openly and it will win every time.

I find countering to be the only effective way to deal with my internet addiction. I'm reminded of the old saying that people on their deathbeds never wish they had spent more time working at the office. To put a modern spin on it, nor do they wish they had watched more TV or spent more time on the internet.

Getting it all to work – a word about routine

"If you were to meet the version of yourself that has reached full potential, what kind of habits would have been developed?" – Derek Doepker

When we retire we are suddenly left without routine. Like all the anticipated joys of retirement, having totally free days can become a millstone without some sort of imposed order.

We need routine in our lives but when we retire it doesn't have to be too rigid.

I love free days, but I do strive to incorporate some gentle, flexible routine into my time simply because having no structure can be frustrating and depressing. It's hard to get much accomplished without at least a smidgeon of discipline.

I start my ideal day with meditation, tea, and some inspirational reading. Walking around on the grass with the dogs. Then breakfast and getting dressed before I hit the computer. A few hours of work. Doing something about lunch. Then more work until sunset. I don't work in the evening. Walk the dogs. Some Netflix, bed.

That would be a typical day if I were at home. Bliss. But of course, very few days are actually like that. I meet friends, have meetings, classes and stuff. But I keep to the plan as much as possible. It gives me a default strategy.

Create a routine for yourself. Imagine an ideal day, an ideal week. What would you do and when? Who with? That's all it takes. It's not complicated.

Here is another easy habit that works well for me. In the morning while still lolling in bed, I decide what I would like to accomplish that day. I imagine myself doing the all the things I want to achieve. I fast forward to the end of the day and notice how good it feels to have done all those things.

Then I set about filling my day with the activities I need to do to accomplish those goals. I still manage to waste a lot of time of course, because I'm an expert at timewasting, but I don't do it quite so much, because I'm filling my time with better things. I feel like I've *earned* my TV time at the end of the day, and that's nice.

Practice a few countering activities every day for at least five minutes. Set yourself a thirty-day challenge to get a new muscle working, a new habit ingrained. That's all. Seriously, I can do it, so you can too.

Physical clutter

"Discipline is the bridge between goals and accomplishment." – Jim Rohn

This section will be short. The simple truth is that the less clutter – mental or physical – that we have in our lives, the easier it will be to find what we want and love doing and the less likely we are to get the blues. Seriously. Clean out a closet, throw away some clothes, give away some knick-knacks and I promise you will not be able to sustain a bad mood. It just feels so good to get rid of stuff!

Clear out, downsize, and get rid of anything that you are no longer using. If you haven't used something in a year, give it away. Clear out your kitchen. Do you really need all those plates? When was the last time you entertained? You need all that space filler that is never used on a day-to-day basis?

Get rid of condiments that are five years old, old salad dressing bottles, give away sheets and towels you don't use; sheets that fit beds you no longer have. Get rid of half of your clothes. You know you don't wear them. That green jacket that looks so cute but doesn't ever go with anything? Those blouses with buttons when you only wear knit tops now? Those old business suits? (Honestly, for years I kept an old suit from my training days in the 90s in England. I thought, what if I need a business suit one day? I didn't and I won't. It's gone now.)

Papers, documents. Go through them and throw out EVERY ONE you don't or won't ever need. Keep only essentials. Touch every piece of paper and decide if you will ever look at it again. Books? Forget it. You have a Kindle now, right? Do you ever read those books? Give away the ones you know you will never read and keep the ones that you will.

I confess I still have old training notes from my stint as a business and personal development trainer in the 90s. But, thing is, I run workshops here in Mexico and I do use the notes from time to time, if only to spark ideas. So I keep them.

Learn to live lean, small, compact, tight, and frugal. This will affect your spirit as well as your wallet. Nobody is quite sure why, but de-cluttering your environment banishes stress in quite miraculous ways.

If you want super inspiration on de-cluttering then Marie Kondo's, *The Life-changing Magic of Tidying Up* is a must. This book has taken over the internet like a storm and is quoted everywhere. You can find it on Amazon and YouTube. I don't often go crazy over books on clearing up, but this one is different.

I'm not a naturally tidy person (does that surprise you?) but this book has inspired me to clear out my house and now it feels calm and serene and I'm much more productive. Also, when I started tidying and giving stuff away, money started flowing into my life from all sorts of sources. Of course most of the Law of Attraction folk will tell you this will happen, and I confess it does sound a bit woo-woo. But it has happened for me. Not just money, but lots of other really cool things have come into my life. As a result I'm a fanatic de-clutterer now. I'm a believer.

Homework

- Cut down on your mental clutter via technology by using at least one or two of the methods listed earlier in the chapter. No need for cold turkey, just cut back.

- Do it for five minutes a day for 30 days.

- Cut down on physical clutter by clearing out your environment.

- Incorporate some easy routines into your day.

- Sit back and notice how much happier you feel.

Modern Problem: too much mental clutter, caused by too much technological input. A modern problem indeed, in fact an epidemic. Our overheated brains cannot cope; we're not evolved to deal with all this technology. It makes us depressed, blue and overwhelmed. *Retirement Pitfall #4.*

Old-fashioned Solution: learn how to use the delete button. Learn how to power down and turn off the computer. Your Mom and Dad coped perfectly well without computers and cell phones. Cut back on your usage.

Your Gran would say go outside, take a walk, and clear your head. Listen to the birds sing and watch the sunset.

Postscript

It's weird how life works sometimes. When we focus intensely on something all kinds of evidence seems to mysteriously appear to reinforce our thoughts.

While I was writing this chapter a few days ago a post came up on my Facebook newsfeed about how silence can actually make our brains grow.

"A 2013 study on mice published in the journal Brain, Structure and Function *used differed types of noise and silence and monitored the effect the sound and silence had on the brains of the mice…*

The scientists discovered that when the mice were exposed to two hours of silence per day they developed new cells in the hippocampus. The hippocampus is a region of the brain associated with memory, emotion and learning.

The growth of new cells in the brain does not necessarily translate to tangible health benefits. However, in this instance, researcher Imke Kirste says that the cells appeared to become functioning neurons."

Can you imagine the implications of this? What if by observing silence every day, we can become more intelligent, prevent dementia, and protect ourselves from Alzheimer's? What if this could make us happier, more serene, more focused, less prone to depression? Spiritual masters and gurus have been telling us this for millennia and we've listened to a certain extent. Now science is beginning to tell us the same thing.

Let's pay attention.

That evening I received an email from a good friend in California whom I had been trying to contact. This is what she wrote:

"SO good to hear your voice in your email…I had no internet for five days! It was the best thing that could have happened. It's the answer to finding happiness. I tell you Margaret…the internet can be our undoing!"

That evening I was so inspired I went to bed without my computer for the first time in about five years. I slept like a log.

Chapter 5
Retirement is Just
the Beginning

"I do know what bliss is: that deep sense of being present,
of doing what you absolutely must do to be yourself."
– Joseph Campbell

I really don't like the word retirement. It conjures up a vision of a horse being put out to pasture – no use to anyone anymore, tired and old. At first it kicks up its heels in joy at not having to pull that carriage anymore...then eats grass until it dies. Who wants that?

HOW TO BEAT THE RETIREMENT BLUES

Why should we retire? I'm pretty sure in many parts of the world the concept is unheard of. People don't retire, they just change the type of work they are doing. It's a modern, industrialized world concept. Sure, at some point we all want to stop working full time and slow down. If we have the finances we may want to opt out of the rat race altogether and do something completely different. But the idea of not working at all, of just eating grass until we die…well no wonder we get the blues! It's just not natural.

Finding *flow* – joy, satisfaction and fulfillment – requires identifying areas where you have mastery or at least a minimum level of skill. I was confronted with an interesting lesson about skill and mastery back in the 1990s, which humbled me and also sowed the seeds for finding my own *flow* later in life.

An interesting visit to an ex-Soviet satellite

I was visiting a friend who was living in the Republic of Georgia, the ex-Soviet satellite bordering Turkey and Azerbaijan – not the southern state where I was born. My friend who had gone there to work for a few years had invited me to come see her, and I thought it would be an interesting place to visit. Certainly off the beaten path of touristy spots I was used to. My friend was working with Georgian youth on various projects.

The experience was eye-opening in a number of ways, but none so much as in the following story.

One evening we had a meeting with a group of teenagers in a rather desolate public hall in Gori, the town where Stalin was born. Gori had a strange vibe. The influence of its most infamous son hangs over the town like a pall. Or maybe that was just my imagination.

The evening meeting was meant to be a social occasion, but there seemed to be no preparations in hand and little food or drink visible. What happened next was akin to feeding the five thousand with a basket of loaves and fishes.

From out of nowhere and seemingly out of nothing a party began. With almost no kitchen utensils or utilities, food was prepared and a feast was offered. Then music and dancing began with instruments magically appearing from somewhere. The entertainment was superb, and when the party was over everything was cleaned up and put away quickly.

Remember folks, teenagers hosted this event. Most of these kids spoke more than one language and some had fluency in several. It was an impressive display of talent and know-how on several levels.

What struck me was this: every young person there had skills in preparing and cooking food for a crowd, playing an instrument to a competent level, and dancing and singing abilities. Plus they knew how to tidy up after themselves. I was spellbound. I do not think I had ever witnessed anything quite like that in the modern industrialized countries I was used to.

I felt like a third thumb. I'm not much of cook at the best of times, but in a totally inadequate kitchen, without all my utensils and cookbooks, forget it. I sat and watched. I can't play an instrument although I did take piano lessons back in the distant past. My dancing is American style disco, which is cringe worthy at the best of times.

HOW TO BEAT THE RETIREMENT BLUES

What was going on? Here I was, a modern American female, educated, earning a lot of money, arguably from the most advanced country in the world, certainly from among the richest, most privileged, educated, most assertive women in history – and I felt like a complete waste of space!

I was the epitome of the modern American female baby boomer who grew up in the 60s. Like many others in my generation, I eschewed learning domestic skills as being beneath me, and had focused on working for a living and having a career. I had a BA degree but couldn't add two plus two, had somehow managed to avoid learning a second language and didn't know basic statistics.

I'm not exaggerating. Just join me and some of my highly educated American female friends here in San Miguel for lunch. Watch what happens when we try to divide up the bill at the end of the meal. It takes us ages.

What exactly am I good at?

The Georgian teenagers were friendly and curious about what I did for a living. I was a sales and management trainer. How do you explain that? I teach people to sell? Managers to manage? It was vaguely disconcerting.

I seriously wondered if I could survive if my modern comforts were removed from me. These kids certainly could. I panicked when the electricity went out for the evening. These kids frequently had to do without electricity for weeks on end.

I had the uncomfortable feeling I wasn't very good at anything useful. It was a chastening experience. What could I learn from this? I felt spoiled and privileged – an evolutionary anomaly. I'm not sure you would want me on your team in the aftermath of the apocalypse.

These kids seemed so well rounded and I was in awe of them – they could do everything. Maybe they had to in order to survive and nobody else was going to do it for them.

It seems that in the industrialized nations we tend to focus most of our education and study on careers. We are very specialized. We are good at our jobs and know how to make money better than anyone. And look at some of the jobs that make tons of money – real estate, insurance selling, business training, hedge fund managing, stockbroking, management consulting. Weird modern careers. Try to explain management consulting in an intelligible way to someone who has never heard of it.

This specialization may be the reason some find themselves in retirement, like Shaquille O'Neal, with nothing much to do other than watch afternoon TV. Ouch. They are so highly trained in one area that they feel lost at sea when they don't have that area to work in anymore.

But hey, there's good news! Specializing can be a boon

Look around you at the retired people who are having the most fun. What are they doing? Lying on the couch watching TV? No way, Jose. They shape a new life based on their old careers. They get creative and figure out how to do something useful, building on what has gone before.

The happiest ex-professional sports people are those who use their skills to create new careers modeled around their sport. John

HOW TO BEAT THE RETIREMENT BLUES

McEnroe exploited his expertise and fame in tennis and has built an empire of sports consulting and commentating; he is obviously totally enjoying himself. Heidi Klum and Tyra Banks used their modeling careers to create enormously popular TV shows and become TV personalities. They're both having fun.

But you don't have to be somebody rich and famous to start a new career. Ordinary retired people write interesting books based on their knowledge and experience. They mentor. They open shops. They consult. They teach.

It dawned on me that now I was retired I could do the same thing – I had the chance to really drill down and hone my motley collection of abilities. I could use what I had learned and frame something new out of those experiences and skills.

One of the causes of the retirement blues is the feeling that your whole working life has been a waste of time. It doesn't need to be. You can use everything you've learned over the years to create something new and magnificent.

I now had time to ponder what message I had, what I could help others with. Was coaching really my thing?

I could work on my skills as a therapist and become an expert in my field. I tweaked some techniques and made up others that work really well. I went to some workshops. My confidence began to grow.

I had the luxury to really work on my niche in coaching and writing. Could I teach others? What did I have to offer?

Who was my natural audience? How about baby boomers, specifically rebellious old hippies like myself? Check.

What was my theme? How about surviving transitions? Helping people in retirement? Check.

I had time and space in my life to figure this stuff out...and it was so much fun! I attended seminars in northern California among the Redwoods. I bought every book on every subject that struck my fancy. I went back and did some more hypnotherapy training and blissed out for two weeks. I did a course on Shamanism and talked to trees. I was having a terrific time and the blues flew out the window. I got too busy for them to flourish.

Retirement gives you the luxury and leisure of space and time.

Hello? Was this what retirement should be about? Rather than the end of work, what if it could be the beginning of excellence? Time to specialize; to become expert in areas you love and that put you in flow. Time to become a source of wisdom for those who are younger. What could be better? Isn't this what we really want?

Retirement can be when you really can bring together years of experience and life-long learning to make a true contribution to the world. What a waste to spend that time goofing off or playing on the internet.

Wake up that Retirement Rebel! This is what it's all about!

Your unique contribution

To get myself out of the doldrums and sailing again, I had to ask myself some stark questions: *What am I good at? What skills do I have? What can I contribute to the world that nobody else can?* These questions are tough, but they push you to find your voice. There is not another you, with your confluence of experience, personality, and talents.

Do this:

- Make an honest list of all the things you can do – everything – and you will be pleasantly surprised at the mastery you have in unexpected places. I'm serious – write a list. This can be quite a game changer.

- Next, put a star by the things you love to do. Mark through what you don't love. Which items make your pulse race?

- Now put a skill rating of 1-5, with 1 being nah and 5 being pretty darn good, next to the things that spark joy in you.

- Mark through anything not starred or rated at least a 3. You don't need them. You don't like them and you aren't any good at them. Bye bye.

What you are left with is what you love to do and that you have some skill in doing. Focus on these. What do they point you to? What work and what service?

Now imagine and dream about what new retirement career you can build on this. It doesn't have to earn money of course. It can be for one day a week. It can be that animal charity you've always wanted to start, or opening a school for indigenous children. What is going to really get you excited about life again?

Getting your life to work, when you don't have to

I got busy doing this when I realized that retirement wasn't working for me. I needed to get working again if I wanted my life to work.

The areas I rated highest on my list were in personal development. I love exploring new ideas about what makes us tick and how to get our lives back on track. All the challenges I was going through. (*Seeker* archetype)

I love sharing those ideas with others. (*Teacher* archetype)

I began spending half my time reading, thinking, mulling over new ideas and self-help techniques, and the other half channeling what I had learned into books, blogs, seminars and coaching. I'm having the best time ever! And I'm earning money again too, which is nice. I've built a new career – a relaxed semi-retirement affair– based on my old one.

I still have my little addictions, but hey, nobody's perfect. An hour or two of Netflix a night never hurt anybody. I still goof around a lot on Facebook way too much, but so what. I'm doing other stuff now to balance it out.

Maybe you can cook, bake, run an online business, design book covers, get social media to work for you, have entrepreneurial skills, love marketing, can teach accounting to dummies, paint signs, do psychic healing – the list is endless.

What can you become expert in? What skills and experience do you have that the world needs? What challenges and setbacks have you overcome that you can help others with? What mode can you use to help them?

Be prepared for those Retirement Pitfalls – travel light and stay alert

Start by **clearing out old emotions and stories** from your past. It's time to re-invent your life: if you are unconsciously clinging to the past you won't be able to move on. So bring it all out, acknowledge what you are missing and grieve, validate, celebrate. Next, push the delete button. You don't need it anymore. Overboard, gone, moving on, thanks.

Then set about **clearing out some of your choices of what to do with your life**. Just winnow them down. You won't lose anything but will gain a lot of clarity. We all get clogged up, stuffed, overfed with too many opportunities and options. Chuck some of them down the hatch and cross them off your list.

Clear out all those things you feel are expected of you but you don't want to do. Pull the plug; watch that bilge drain away. Nice...

Stop doing things you don't want to do. This is your time now.

Meanwhile, **clear out your environment, get rid of clutter**, downsize and liberate yourself from half your stuff. You want to be lean and mean, fighting fit and ready for action. You don't need to be collecting any more stuff in your life. In fact, if you want clarity and joy, then go ahead and clear out. Leave it all on the docks. You sail better when you sail lighter.

Ah, now, before you set off, make time to sit by a tree, walk barefoot on the grass, bask in the early morning sun, and play with your dog. (If you don't have a dog or cat then go get one.) Learn how to log out and shut down your computer. Power down the phone and sit in silence. Allow your mind to cool down and regrow those brain cells.

This will give you the space you need to redesign your life.

This is your time to really discover yourself, find your true purpose and make a contribution. Nobody has your experience and skills. Sign up for that seminar in Santa Fe. Go to that retreat in Sedona. Go camping in the desert. (Well, maybe not that last one...)

Retirement is just the beginning. You're not meant to stop living your life, you're meant to take time out to regroup and reinvent your life. It's a chance to get really good at what you love. Your time is now.

Kick that sleeping *Retirement Rebel/Pirate* off the couch. Hoist those sails and catch the wind!

Smooth sailing!

Did you like what you just read?

If so I would LOVE and APPRECIATE a nice review. Reviews help indie authors more than you can possibly imagine. I will even buy you lunch if you're ever in San Miguel de Allende, Mexico.

That's a promise—tacos on me.

Just go to the page on amazon.com for ***The Retirement Rebel*** and click on reviews – or use this link:

getbook.at/retirement-rebel

Please download my FREE e-book

The Rebellious Entrepreneur
5 crucial steps to help you establish yourself profess-ionally and make a success of your business or practice.

Find your voice, your identity, and position yourself in the marketplace.

Get it now!

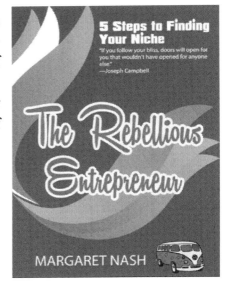

www.margaretnashcoach.com/5-steps

Would you like to work online with Margaret Nash?

Professional, affordable, first class Life–Coaching that will guarantee results in your life and work. Watch your productivity soar with as you create good work habits, motivational goals, and strategies for manifesting the life you want.

Find out more about her online *Life-Coaching* at

www.margaretnashcoach.com/life-coaching

We use Facebook Messenger or Zoom. No video.
Pay for each session via PayPal—simple, easy, quick.
Check it out

www.margaretnashcoach.com/life-coaching

What's your next big step in life? Try *Life-Coaching* and make it happen!

About Margaret Nash

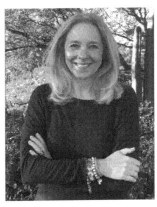

Margaret Nash lives and works as a writer, life coach, seminar leader, wife, dog owner, and friend who will lunch at the drop of a hat, in San Miguel de Allende in the Central Highlands of Mexico.

She grew up in Alabama, in the 1960s, and after college visited England and stayed for three decades.

Margaret's blog, and her books, *Rebellious Aging, Drop the Drama! How to Get Along With Everybody, All the Time, The Retirement Rebel, Artful Assertiveness Skills for Women,* and *Follow the Trail of Your Spirit*, deal with the themes of aging well, surviving transitions, and finding your niche in life in your 50s, 60s, and beyond.

Her demographic is the *rebel/hippie at heart/fiercely independent free spirit* facing major life changes and determined to age in the coolest way possible.

Margaret is a Master Practitioner & Trainer/Coach in NLP, Hypnosis and Time-line Therapy. She has been in practice for 17 years.

She is a certified aging brat/skeptic/seeker/searcher— and definitely a hippie at heart.

www.margaretnashcoach.com

If you enjoyed *The Retirement Rebel*, you will love Margaret's book *Rebellious Aging: A Self-Help guide for the Old Hippie at Heart.*

Aging can be fun! You just need to awaken your Rebel and survive those transitions.

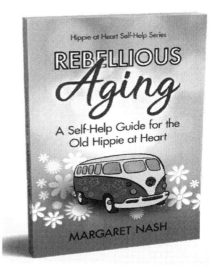

This book is a motivational, self-help guide for you if you are a hippie at heart— in other words unconventional, fiercely independent and a bit of a rebel— determined to find your niche in life and enjoy yourself as you grow older.

It is a book about transitions; the transitions of life that sometimes hit you hard, like retirement, kids leaving home, divorce, relocation … or waking up one morning and realizing you are no longer a spring chicken.

So hop into your hippie van and take a Hero's Journey down into your subconscious mind to find your true self, your authentic voice, and practical and effective ways to survive all the changes piling up on you.

The methods and processes included here can't be found in the doctor's office or on a psychoanalyst's couch. They are unorthodox and will appeal to the hippie in you. But don't be mislead—this book contains effective life-coaching tips and techniques for personal inner transformation.

Download your kindle copy today:

getbook.at/rebellious-aging

You may also enjoy *Drop the Drama! How to Get Along With Everybody, All the Time* also by Margaret Nash, available in kindle and paperback on Amazon.

Do You Want a Drama Free Life? Then Drop the Drama!

Are you tired of squabbling, trying to make amends with people you have offended, or clearing up misunderstandings? Sick of dealing with your own hurt feelings?

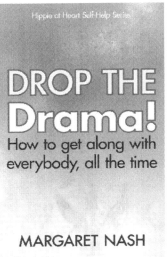

Look no further. Read this book!

Adopt these skills and rock all relationships!

It's possible to turn over a new leaf right now. You absolutely can learn how to *get along with everybody, all the time*, no matter who you are, how cantankerous, and despite any past relationship disasters.

But you are going to have to learn to play nice, even when you don't feel like it. You can do this.

So I invite you to absorb this book and put your nose to the grindstone practicing the **six social skills** outlined—until they become second nature. You will be glad you did.

In this easy to read self-help guide:

- Be introduced to the ***Most Useful Relationship Technique Ever in the History of the Universe*** (no hyperbole!).

- Find out how to avoid being the ***least popular type of person***.

- Discover your **personality style** and how you can use it to get along with everybody.

- Learn the *secret sauce* to fabulous relationships.

These skills are culled from the cutting-edge life enhancing techniques of **Neuro-linguistic Programming**, along with a plethora of tried and true skills from Don Miguel Ruiz to Dale Carnegie to Eckhart Tolle.

Once you 'get' them everything will become easier and you will create **stress-free, ruffled-feather-free relationships** with everyone in your life. That's a promise!

Download your kindle copy today:

getbook.at/drop-drama

Ladies, if you suffer from not being heard or taken seriously, *Artful Assertiveness Skills for Women,* **By Margaret Nash** may be the book for you!

Attention Ladies of all ages, shapes, sizes, and personalities! Would you like to learn how to stand up for yourself, gain respect, and handle *every* situation with calm assurance and authority? Yes?

Then you need to read this book! It's time for **Assertiveness Boot Camp** and this book is your self-help Boot Camp Guide.

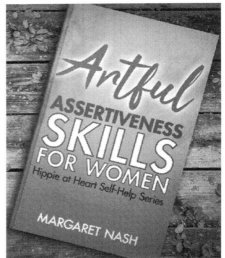

So pull on your fatigues, lace up your boots, and let's get to work!

Welcome to *Artful Assertiveness Skills for Women.* Here you will learn the basic rules of assertiveness:

- Learn how to say no, artfully and effectively without anyone getting upset.

- Define and protect your boundaries without anyone noticing.

- Project a calm, confident energy that will make the Dog Whisperer jealous.

- Shut down bullies and passive-aggressive, catty types with style and wit.

- Learn the body language that will ensure you are listened to and taken seriously. Avoid these seven common mistakes.

- Practice the best way to complain about bad service.

- Discover how to keep yourself safe both physically and emotionally.

But it takes some work! You'll going to learn some awesome and artful responses that will just trip off your tongue the next time you are upset, ignored, or challenged.

You will also pick up some very useful body language tips that may save your bacon one day and learn the secret of how to exude an energy that makes people sit up, listen and treat you with respect.

This self-help guide is fun, easy to read and will keep you entertained with real life stories to illustrate how assertiveness works, or doesn't work.

You'll get Boot Camp homework—phrases and sentences to practice—after every chapter. You can literally just copy down useful responses and use them verbatim.

It's different from other assertiveness training—it really emphasizes the artful bit— which means you always come across as natural, friendly and relaxed while still getting the respect you deserve.

This is the 4th book in the *Hippie at Heart Self-help Series* by Margaret Nash, Life-Coach, Business Trainer, NLP Master Practitioner, self-help writer, aging brat, hippie at heart…as she shares her years of experience with clients, family, friends, dogs and cats, honing her assertiveness skills. (OK, it didn't work with the cats.)

What people are saying about Artful Assertiveness Skills for Women:

"This book has so much valuable advice on modern life for the modern woman. You'll learn how to handle difficult people and stressful situations --without stress! Margaret Nash offers a

refreshing perspective on women's issues in the workplace and in day-to-day interactions." SP Ericson

"This is a timely book. The rise of the **MeToo** *movement spawns stories indicating far too many women lack skills in assertiveness. Standing up in situations where power is the undercurrent is hard. This is an important book. Nash's chapter on creating boundaries and another on 'combat training' made this an especially good read. Buy this for you.... and your daughters."* Barbara Pagano

"I teach assertiveness skills in my business and LOVE this book! Margaret provides clear stories and solutions so that reader's assertiveness muscles will get bigger and bigger as they flex their healthy, compassionate, courageous power." Trina

"This book delivers ~ chapter after chapter after chapter ~ and percolates along with such an upbeat and companionable delivery that the reader cannot help but gain an infusion of the Artful Assertiveness Skills author Margaret Nash promises!"

"While she employs such yang training metaphors as "Boot Camp" and "Test Pilots," she does so in a manner that serves the yin value of relationship: attaining these aptitudes not for "power-over" ends, but in order to cultivate win-win accord. As this book is written with women in mind, this is most satisfactory in terms of Jungian Psychology, which teaches that a woman's animus, or masculine dimension, is there to serve her womanly nature." Mary Trainor-Brigham

"Up 'til now I have been the kind of woman who usually said 'yes' when I really meant 'no'! Reading Margaret Nash's book has encouraged me to be more authentic with my real feelings with a new courage to speak my truth without being abrasive.

Having been a 'nice girl' all of my life, I was a natural people pleaser and generally said what people wanted to hear.

I'm very encouraged after reading and practicing 'Artful Assertiveness Skills for Women' and I'm enjoying this newfound

freedom... my communication skills have become more forthright. I have used many of the suggestions in this book ... especially the one of asking questions like, 'now why would you say that?' or 'What do you mean by that comment?' A question seems to stop an aggressive person in their tracks and the dynamic quickly changes. So far, I've not offended any of my friends and have a much better relationship with my employee who thought she was boss! I highly recommend." Sabrina

"This book lays out a concise, easy plan or boot camp for improving daily interactions with every person you encounter. With lists of exact actions & dialogues to facilitate desired outcomes, I wasn't surprised the author has spent much of her career as a life coach. It doesn't read like a self-help book, but more as an action plan to guide us toward results. Easy & interesting read. Wish I had access to this at age 20 instead of 50!" Krista Yarnell

"Bought at book at the local library for my 25 year old daughter and she loved it! Never too early or late to start learning this stuff!" Joseph Toone

Download your kindle copy today:

getbook.at/artful-assertiveness

If you wonder what life is all about and what your role is, you will love Margaret's latest book, *Follow the Trail of Your Spirit: A Step-by-Step Guide to Finding Life Purpose.* You will never need another book on finding purpose!

Follow the Trail of Your Spirit is a fast-paced, easy-to-read, down-to-earth life-coaching guide to finding purpose, meaningful activity, and your perfect career.

Wouldn't it be nice if you could find productive, satisfying, and fulfilling things to do, whether at work or simply hanging out at home, by just answering 10 questions?

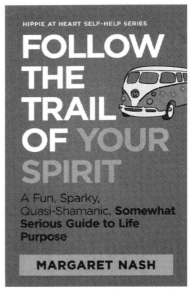

You can! Just by reading this book! No more feeling frustrated, disappointed in yourself, or suffering that nagging sense you are missing out on something big. You can start enjoying life with the first chapter.

Readers have reported feeling more focused, mindful, and motivated, and love the humor, fresh ideas, and use of personal stories in the book. Also the section on Archetypes and how they can help you find your purpose is cited as intriguing and useful.

Margaret Nash has been a successful Life Coach, Business Trainer, and NLP Seminar Leader for over 20 years and is the author of 5 coaching books in her *Hippie-at-Heart Self-Help Series*—all available on Amazon.

She will take you on her personal journey from Alabama to England to Mexico searching for meaning, purpose, and her

professional identity. She will share with you her discoveries along the way as well as real life stories from her many clients.

She found out

- Why 'follow your passion' could be **the worst advice ever**

- The **only 10 life coaching questions** you'll ever need to discover exactly what you're looking for

- How your worst **mistakes and failures are a goldmine** you can transform into your greatest success

- There's always room for you, and **what you have to offer counts** to someone. Find your place in the world. You count.

Follow the Trail of Your Spirit is served up with a touch of mysticism, a dash of inspiration, and a taste of shamanism.

Grab your copy today!

getbook.at/follow-trail

Notes

Inspirations

Notes

Inspirations

Notes

Inspirations

Notes

Inspirations

Made in the USA
Las Vegas, NV
14 October 2021